——EXERCISE——• SETS •—— REPS AND DONE! ——•

ello.

here is no need for me to explain the boxes for Sets, Reps and Done…. You know hat you're doing there!

owever! I would like to explain the **Small Dots** on the outside f each page and the "**Best Increase**" box.

Dependent on your routine and days in the gym, you on't want to use one page per workout and waste space. o the dots are your "Date Link Line" as shown here.

ink the boxes to indicate one session in the gym and vrite the day above the line.

ven if the last three exercise boxes are spare from any vork out, you can link them to the next page and so on.

Best weight increase….. As it says on the tin!

When you increase your weight through your sets, write the best increase in weight as a marker for future gains in weight. This way you can refer to it down the line to see your increase performance.

Thanks for purchasing this Training Journal and I hope it works well for you. Feedback s good for me so I can improve future editions, so all comments are welcome.

Other Journals in the our range include High Intensity Tracker, Arm Blast and Bulk Up. Have a good workout!

www.the**body**plan**plus**.com

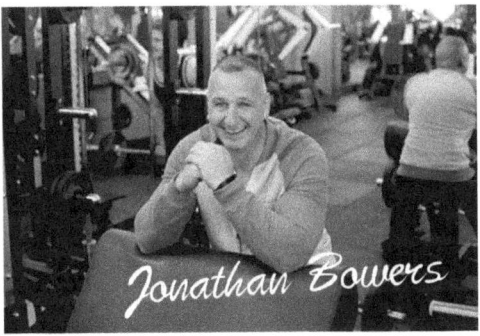

Jonathan Bowers

Author: Jonathan Bowers
Copyright 2015
The Body Plan Plus ™

EXERCISE	SETS	REPS AND DONE!				
		REPS ☐	REPS ☐	REPS ☐	REPS ☐	REPS ☐
BEST INCREASE WEIGHT						
		REPS ☐	REPS ☐	REPS ☐	REPS ☐	REPS ☐
BEST INCREASE WEIGHT						
		REPS ☐	REPS ☐	REPS ☐	REPS ☐	REPS ☐
BEST INCREASE WEIGHT						
		REPS ☐	REPS ☐	REPS ☐	REPS ☐	REPS ☐
BEST INCREASE WEIGHT						
		REPS ☐	REPS ☐	REPS ☐	REPS ☐	REPS ☐
BEST INCREASE WEIGHT						
		REPS ☐	REPS ☐	REPS ☐	REPS ☐	REPS ☐
BEST INCREASE WEIGHT						
		REPS ☐	REPS ☐	REPS ☐	REPS ☐	REPS ☐
BEST INCREASE WEIGHT						
		REPS ☐	REPS ☐	REPS ☐	REPS ☐	REPS ☐
BEST INCREASE WEIGHT						
		REPS ☐	REPS ☐	REPS ☐	REPS ☐	REPS ☐
BEST INCREASE WEIGHT						
		REPS ☐	REPS ☐	REPS ☐	REPS ☐	REPS ☐
BEST INCREASE WEIGHT						
		REPS ☐	REPS ☐	REPS ☐	REPS ☐	REPS ☐
BEST INCREASE WEIGHT						

EXERCISE ———— SETS ———— REPS AND DONE! ————

	SETS	REPS ✓	REPS ✓	REPS ✓	REPS ✓	REPS ✓
BEST INCREASE → WEIGHT →						
		REPS ☐	REPS ☐	REPS ☐	REPS ☐	REPS ☐
BEST INCREASE → WEIGHT →						
		REPS ☐	REPS ☐	REPS ☐	REPS ☐	REPS ☐
BEST INCREASE → WEIGHT →						
		REPS ☐	REPS ☐	REPS ☐	REPS ☐	REPS ☐
BEST INCREASE → WEIGHT →						
		REPS ☐	REPS ☐	REPS ☐	REPS ☐	REPS ☐
BEST INCREASE → WEIGHT →						
		REPS ☐	REPS ☐	REPS ☐	REPS ☐	REPS ☐
BEST INCREASE → WEIGHT →						
		REPS ☐	REPS ☐	REPS ☐	REPS ☐	REPS ☐
BEST INCREASE → WEIGHT →						
		REPS ☐	REPS ☐	REPS ☐	REPS ☐	REPS ☐
BEST INCREASE → WEIGHT →						
		REPS ☐	REPS ☐	REPS ☐	REPS ☐	REPS ☐
BEST INCREASE → WEIGHT →						
		REPS ☐	REPS ☐	REPS ☐	REPS ☐	REPS ☐
BEST INCREASE → WEIGHT →						
		REPS ☐	REPS ☐	REPS ☐	REPS ☐	REPS ☐
BEST INCREASE → WEIGHT →						
		REPS ☐	REPS ☐	REPS ☐	REPS ☐	REPS ☐
BEST INCREASE → WEIGHT →						

EXERCISE	SETS	REPS AND DONE!

EXERCISE	SETS	REPS ✓	REPS ✓	REPS ✓	REPS ✓	REPS ✓
	BEST INCREASE WEIGHT					
		REPS	REPS	REPS	REPS	REPS
	BEST INCREASE WEIGHT					
		REPS	REPS	REPS	REPS	REPS
	BEST INCREASE WEIGHT					
		REPS	REPS	REPS	REPS	REPS
	BEST INCREASE WEIGHT					
		REPS	REPS	REPS	REPS	REPS
	BEST INCREASE WEIGHT					
		REPS	REPS	REPS	REPS	REPS
	BEST INCREASE WEIGHT					
		REPS	REPS	REPS	REPS	REPS
	BEST INCREASE WEIGHT					
		REPS	REPS	REPS	REPS	REPS
	BEST INCREASE WEIGHT					
		REPS	REPS	REPS	REPS	REPS
	BEST INCREASE WEIGHT					
		REPS	REPS	REPS	REPS	REPS
	BEST INCREASE WEIGHT					

EXERCISE	SETS	REPS AND DONE!				
		REPS ☑	REPS ☑	REPS ☑	REPS ☑	REPS ☑
BEST INCREASE → WEIGHT →						
		REPS ☐	REPS ☐	REPS ☐	REPS ☐	REPS ☐
BEST INCREASE → WEIGHT →						
		REPS ☐	REPS ☐	REPS ☐	REPS ☐	REPS ☐
BEST INCREASE → WEIGHT →						
		REPS ☐	REPS ☐	REPS ☐	REPS ☐	REPS ☐
BEST INCREASE → WEIGHT →						
		REPS ☐	REPS ☐	REPS ☐	REPS ☐	REPS ☐
BEST INCREASE → WEIGHT →						
		REPS ☐	REPS ☐	REPS ☐	REPS ☐	REPS ☐
BEST INCREASE → WEIGHT →						
		REPS ☐	REPS ☐	REPS ☐	REPS ☐	REPS ☐
BEST INCREASE → WEIGHT →						
		REPS ☐	REPS ☐	REPS ☐	REPS ☐	REPS ☐
BEST INCREASE → WEIGHT →						
		REPS ☐	REPS ☐	REPS ☐	REPS ☐	REPS ☐
BEST INCREASE → WEIGHT →						
		REPS ☐	REPS ☐	REPS ☐	REPS ☐	REPS ☐
BEST INCREASE → WEIGHT →						
		REPS ☐	REPS ☐	REPS ☐	REPS ☐	REPS ☐
BEST INCREASE → WEIGHT →						
		REPS ☐	REPS ☐	REPS ☐	REPS ☐	REPS ☐
BEST INCREASE → WEIGHT →						

EXERCISE	SETS	REPS AND DONE!
		REPS ☐ REPS ☐ REPS ☐ REPS ☐ REPS ☐
BEST INCREASE ◄ WEIGHT ►		
		REPS ☐ REPS ☐ REPS ☐ REPS ☐ REPS ☐
BEST INCREASE ◄ WEIGHT ►		
		REPS ☐ REPS ☐ REPS ☐ REPS ☐ REPS ☐
BEST INCREASE ◄ WEIGHT ►		
		REPS ☐ REPS ☐ REPS ☐ REPS ☐ REPS ☐
BEST INCREASE ◄ WEIGHT ►		
		REPS ☐ REPS ☐ REPS ☐ REPS ☐ REPS ☐
BEST INCREASE ◄ WEIGHT ►		
		REPS ☐ REPS ☐ REPS ☐ REPS ☐ REPS ☐
BEST INCREASE ◄ WEIGHT ►		
		REPS ☐ REPS ☐ REPS ☐ REPS ☐ REPS ☐
BEST INCREASE ◄ WEIGHT ►		
		REPS ☐ REPS ☐ REPS ☐ REPS ☐ REPS ☐
BEST INCREASE ◄ WEIGHT ►		
		REPS ☐ REPS ☐ REPS ☐ REPS ☐ REPS ☐
BEST INCREASE ◄ WEIGHT ►		
		REPS ☐ REPS ☐ REPS ☐ REPS ☐ REPS ☐
BEST INCREASE ◄ WEIGHT ►		

EXERCISE ———— SETS ———— REPS AND DONE! ————

EXERCISE	SETS	REPS ✓	REPS ✓	REPS ✓	REPS ✓	REPS ✓
BEST INCREASE → WEIGHT →						
		REPS	REPS	REPS	REPS	REPS
BEST INCREASE → WEIGHT →						
		REPS	REPS	REPS	REPS	REPS
BEST INCREASE → WEIGHT →						
		REPS	REPS	REPS	REPS	REPS
BEST INCREASE → WEIGHT →						
		REPS	REPS	REPS	REPS	REPS
BEST INCREASE → WEIGHT →						
		REPS	REPS	REPS	REPS	REPS
BEST INCREASE → WEIGHT →						
		REPS	REPS	REPS	REPS	REPS
BEST INCREASE → WEIGHT →						
		REPS	REPS	REPS	REPS	REPS
BEST INCREASE → WEIGHT →						
		REPS	REPS	REPS	REPS	REPS
BEST INCREASE → WEIGHT →						
		REPS	REPS	REPS	REPS	REPS
BEST INCREASE → WEIGHT →						
		REPS	REPS	REPS	REPS	REPS
BEST INCREASE → WEIGHT →						
		REPS	REPS	REPS	REPS	REPS
BEST INCREASE → WEIGHT →						

EXERCISE	SETS	REPS AND DONE!				
		REPS ☐	REPS ☐	REPS ☐	REPS ☐	REPS ☐
☐ BEST INCREASE ◄ WEIGHT ►						
		REPS ☐	REPS ☐	REPS ☐	REPS ☐	REPS ☐
☐ BEST INCREASE ◄ WEIGHT ►						
		REPS ☐	REPS ☐	REPS ☐	REPS ☐	REPS ☐
☐ BEST INCREASE ◄ WEIGHT ►						
		REPS ☐	REPS ☐	REPS ☐	REPS ☐	REPS ☐
☐ BEST INCREASE ◄ WEIGHT ►						
		REPS ☐	REPS ☐	REPS ☐	REPS ☐	REPS ☐
☐ BEST INCREASE ◄ WEIGHT ►						
		REPS ☐	REPS ☐	REPS ☐	REPS ☐	REPS ☐
☐ BEST INCREASE ◄ WEIGHT ►						
		REPS ☐	REPS ☐	REPS ☐	REPS ☐	REPS ☐
☐ BEST INCREASE ◄ WEIGHT ►						
		REPS ☐	REPS ☐	REPS ☐	REPS ☐	REPS ☐
☐ BEST INCREASE ◄ WEIGHT ►						
		REPS ☐	REPS ☐	REPS ☐	REPS ☐	REPS ☐
☐ BEST INCREASE ◄ WEIGHT ►						
		REPS ☐	REPS ☐	REPS ☐	REPS ☐	REPS ☐
☐ BEST INCREASE ◄ WEIGHT ►						
		REPS ☐	REPS ☐	REPS ☐	REPS ☐	REPS ☐
☐ BEST INCREASE ◄ WEIGHT ►						

EXERCISE	SETS	REPS AND DONE!
		REPS ✓	REPS ✓	REPS ✓	REPS ✓	REPS ✓
BEST INCREASE WEIGHT						
		REPS	REPS	REPS	REPS	REPS
BEST INCREASE WEIGHT						
		REPS	REPS	REPS	REPS	REPS
BEST INCREASE WEIGHT						
		REPS	REPS	REPS	REPS	REPS
BEST INCREASE WEIGHT						
		REPS	REPS	REPS	REPS	REPS
BEST INCREASE WEIGHT						
		REPS	REPS	REPS	REPS	REPS
BEST INCREASE WEIGHT						
		REPS	REPS	REPS	REPS	REPS
BEST INCREASE WEIGHT						
		REPS	REPS	REPS	REPS	REPS
BEST INCREASE WEIGHT						
		REPS	REPS	REPS	REPS	REPS
BEST INCREASE WEIGHT						
		REPS	REPS	REPS	REPS	REPS
BEST INCREASE WEIGHT						
		REPS	REPS	REPS	REPS	REPS
BEST INCREASE WEIGHT						
		REPS	REPS	REPS	REPS	REPS
BEST INCREASE WEIGHT						

		REPS ☐	REPS ☐	REPS ☐	REPS ☐	REPS ☐
BEST INCREASE WEIGHT						
		REPS ☐	REPS ☐	REPS ☐	REPS ☐	REPS ☐
BEST INCREASE WEIGHT						
		REPS ☐	REPS ☐	REPS ☐	REPS ☐	REPS ☐
BEST INCREASE WEIGHT						
		REPS ☐	REPS ☐	REPS ☐	REPS ☐	REPS ☐
BEST INCREASE WEIGHT						
		REPS ☐	REPS ☐	REPS ☐	REPS ☐	REPS ☐
BEST INCREASE WEIGHT						
		REPS ☐	REPS ☐	REPS ☐	REPS ☐	REPS ☐
BEST INCREASE WEIGHT						
		REPS ☐	REPS ☐	REPS ☐	REPS ☐	REPS ☐
BEST INCREASE WEIGHT						
		REPS ☐	REPS ☐	REPS ☐	REPS ☐	REPS ☐
BEST INCREASE WEIGHT						
		REPS ☐	REPS ☐	REPS ☐	REPS ☐	REPS ☐
BEST INCREASE WEIGHT						

EXERCISE	SETS	REPS AND DONE!				
		REPS ✔	REPS ✔	REPS ✔	REPS ✔	REPS ✔
BEST INCREASE ← WEIGHT →						
		REPS	REPS	REPS	REPS	REPS
BEST INCREASE ← WEIGHT →						
		REPS	REPS	REPS	REPS	REPS
BEST INCREASE ← WEIGHT →						
		REPS	REPS	REPS	REPS	REPS
BEST INCREASE ← WEIGHT →						
		REPS	REPS	REPS	REPS	REPS
BEST INCREASE ← WEIGHT →						
		REPS	REPS	REPS	REPS	REPS
BEST INCREASE ← WEIGHT →						
		REPS	REPS	REPS	REPS	REPS
BEST INCREASE ← WEIGHT →						
		REPS	REPS	REPS	REPS	REPS
BEST INCREASE ← WEIGHT →						
		REPS	REPS	REPS	REPS	REPS
BEST INCREASE ← WEIGHT →						
		REPS	REPS	REPS	REPS	REPS
BEST INCREASE ← WEIGHT →						
		REPS	REPS	REPS	REPS	REPS
BEST INCREASE ← WEIGHT →						

EXERCISE	SETS	REPS AND DONE!				
		REPS ☐	REPS ☐	REPS ☐	REPS ☐	REPS ☐
BEST INCREASE — WEIGHT						
		REPS ☐	REPS ☐	REPS ☐	REPS ☐	REPS ☐
BEST INCREASE — WEIGHT						
		REPS ☐	REPS ☐	REPS ☐	REPS ☐	REPS ☐
BEST INCREASE — WEIGHT						
		REPS ☐	REPS ☐	REPS ☐	REPS ☐	REPS ☐
BEST INCREASE — WEIGHT						
		REPS ☐	REPS ☐	REPS ☐	REPS ☐	REPS ☐
BEST INCREASE — WEIGHT						
		REPS ☐	REPS ☐	REPS ☐	REPS ☐	REPS ☐
BEST INCREASE — WEIGHT						
		REPS ☐	REPS ☐	REPS ☐	REPS ☐	REPS ☐
BEST INCREASE — WEIGHT						
		REPS ☐	REPS ☐	REPS ☐	REPS ☐	REPS ☐
BEST INCREASE — WEIGHT						
		REPS ☐	REPS ☐	REPS ☐	REPS ☐	REPS ☐
BEST INCREASE — WEIGHT						
		REPS ☐	REPS ☐	REPS ☐	REPS ☐	REPS ☐
BEST INCREASE — WEIGHT						
		REPS ☐	REPS ☐	REPS ☐	REPS ☐	REPS ☐
BEST INCREASE — WEIGHT						

EXERCISE	SETS	REPS ✔	REPS ✔	REPS ✔	REPS ✔	REPS ✔
BEST INCREASE ← WEIGHT →						
		REPS ☐	REPS ☐	REPS ☐	REPS ☐	REPS ☐
BEST INCREASE ← WEIGHT →						
		REPS ☐	REPS ☐	REPS ☐	REPS ☐	REPS ☐
BEST INCREASE ← WEIGHT →						
		REPS ☐	REPS ☐	REPS ☐	REPS ☐	REPS ☐
BEST INCREASE ← WEIGHT →						
		REPS ☐	REPS ☐	REPS ☐	REPS ☐	REPS ☐
BEST INCREASE ← WEIGHT →						
		REPS ☐	REPS ☐	REPS ☐	REPS ☐	REPS ☐
BEST INCREASE ← WEIGHT →						
		REPS ☐	REPS ☐	REPS ☐	REPS ☐	REPS ☐
BEST INCREASE ← WEIGHT →						
		REPS ☐	REPS ☐	REPS ☐	REPS ☐	REPS ☐
BEST INCREASE ← WEIGHT →						
		REPS ☐	REPS ☐	REPS ☐	REPS ☐	REPS ☐
BEST INCREASE ← WEIGHT →						
		REPS ☐	REPS ☐	REPS ☐	REPS ☐	REPS ☐
BEST INCREASE ← WEIGHT →						
		REPS ☐	REPS ☐	REPS ☐	REPS ☐	REPS ☐
BEST INCREASE ← WEIGHT →						
		REPS ☐	REPS ☐	REPS ☐	REPS ☐	REPS ☐
BEST INCREASE ← WEIGHT →						

		REPS ☑	REPS ☑	REPS ☑	REPS ☑	REPS ☑
BEST INCREASE WEIGHT						
		REPS ◯	REPS ◯	REPS ◯	REPS ◯	REPS ◯
BEST INCREASE WEIGHT						
		REPS ◯	REPS ◯	REPS ◯	REPS ◯	REPS ◯
BEST INCREASE WEIGHT						
		REPS ◯	REPS ◯	REPS ◯	REPS ◯	REPS ◯
BEST INCREASE WEIGHT						
		REPS ◯	REPS ◯	REPS ◯	REPS ◯	REPS ◯
BEST INCREASE WEIGHT						
		REPS ◯	REPS ◯	REPS ◯	REPS ◯	REPS ◯
BEST INCREASE WEIGHT						
		REPS ◯	REPS ◯	REPS ◯	REPS ◯	REPS ◯
BEST INCREASE WEIGHT						
		REPS ◯	REPS ◯	REPS ◯	REPS ◯	REPS ◯
BEST INCREASE WEIGHT						
		REPS ◯	REPS ◯	REPS ◯	REPS ◯	REPS ◯
BEST INCREASE WEIGHT						
		REPS ◯	REPS ◯	REPS ◯	REPS ◯	REPS ◯
BEST INCREASE WEIGHT						
		REPS ◯	REPS ◯	REPS ◯	REPS ◯	REPS ◯
BEST INCREASE WEIGHT						

EXERCISE ———— SETS ———— REPS AND DONE! ————

		REPS ✓	REPS ✓	REPS ✓	REPS ✓	REPS ✓
BEST INCREASE WEIGHT						
		REPS	REPS	REPS	REPS	REPS
BEST INCREASE WEIGHT						
		REPS	REPS	REPS	REPS	REPS
BEST INCREASE WEIGHT						
		REPS	REPS	REPS	REPS	REPS
BEST INCREASE WEIGHT						
		REPS	REPS	REPS	REPS	REPS
BEST INCREASE WEIGHT						
		REPS	REPS	REPS	REPS	REPS
BEST INCREASE WEIGHT						
		REPS	REPS	REPS	REPS	REPS
BEST INCREASE WEIGHT						
		REPS	REPS	REPS	REPS	REPS
BEST INCREASE WEIGHT						
		REPS	REPS	REPS	REPS	REPS
BEST INCREASE WEIGHT						
		REPS	REPS	REPS	REPS	REPS
BEST INCREASE WEIGHT						
		REPS	REPS	REPS	REPS	REPS
BEST INCREASE WEIGHT						

		REPS ☐	REPS ☐	REPS ☐	REPS ☐	REPS ☐
BEST INCREASE ← WEIGHT →						
		REPS ☐	REPS ☐	REPS ☐	REPS ☐	REPS ☐
BEST INCREASE ← WEIGHT →						
		REPS ☐	REPS ☐	REPS ☐	REPS ☐	REPS ☐
BEST INCREASE ← WEIGHT →						
		REPS ☐	REPS ☐	REPS ☐	REPS ☐	REPS ☐
BEST INCREASE ← WEIGHT →						
		REPS ☐	REPS ☐	REPS ☐	REPS ☐	REPS ☐
BEST INCREASE ← WEIGHT →						
		REPS ☐	REPS ☐	REPS ☐	REPS ☐	REPS ☐
BEST INCREASE ← WEIGHT →						
		REPS ☐	REPS ☐	REPS ☐	REPS ☐	REPS ☐
BEST INCREASE ← WEIGHT →						
		REPS ☐	REPS ☐	REPS ☐	REPS ☐	REPS ☐
BEST INCREASE ← WEIGHT →						
		REPS ☐	REPS ☐	REPS ☐	REPS ☐	REPS ☐
BEST INCREASE ← WEIGHT →						
		REPS ☐	REPS ☐	REPS ☐	REPS ☐	REPS ☐
BEST INCREASE ← WEIGHT →						

EXERCISE	SETS	REPS ✓	REPS ✓	REPS ✓	REPS ✓	REPS ✓
BEST INCREASE — WEIGHT						
		REPS ⬡	REPS ⬡	REPS ⬡	REPS ⬡	REPS ⬡
BEST INCREASE — WEIGHT						
		REPS ⬡	REPS ⬡	REPS ⬡	REPS ⬡	REPS ⬡
BEST INCREASE — WEIGHT						
		REPS ⬡	REPS ⬡	REPS ⬡	REPS ⬡	REPS ⬡
BEST INCREASE — WEIGHT						
		REPS ⬡	REPS ⬡	REPS ⬡	REPS ⬡	REPS ⬡
BEST INCREASE — WEIGHT						
		REPS ⬡	REPS ⬡	REPS ⬡	REPS ⬡	REPS ⬡
BEST INCREASE — WEIGHT						
		REPS ⬡	REPS ⬡	REPS ⬡	REPS ⬡	REPS ⬡
BEST INCREASE — WEIGHT						
		REPS ⬡	REPS ⬡	REPS ⬡	REPS ⬡	REPS ⬡
BEST INCREASE — WEIGHT						
		REPS ⬡	REPS ⬡	REPS ⬡	REPS ⬡	REPS ⬡
BEST INCREASE — WEIGHT						
		REPS ⬡	REPS ⬡	REPS ⬡	REPS ⬡	REPS ⬡
BEST INCREASE — WEIGHT						
		REPS ⬡	REPS ⬡	REPS ⬡	REPS ⬡	REPS ⬡
BEST INCREASE — WEIGHT						

EXERCISE	SETS	REPS AND DONE!
		REPS ☐ REPS ☐ REPS ☐ REPS ☐ REPS ☐
☐ BEST INCREASE WEIGHT		
		REPS ☐ REPS ☐ REPS ☐ REPS ☐ REPS ☐
☐ BEST INCREASE WEIGHT		
		REPS ☐ REPS ☐ REPS ☐ REPS ☐ REPS ☐
☐ BEST INCREASE WEIGHT		
		REPS ☐ REPS ☐ REPS ☐ REPS ☐ REPS ☐
☐ BEST INCREASE WEIGHT		
		REPS ☐ REPS ☐ REPS ☐ REPS ☐ REPS ☐
☐ BEST INCREASE WEIGHT		
		REPS ☐ REPS ☐ REPS ☐ REPS ☐ REPS ☐
☐ BEST INCREASE WEIGHT		
		REPS ☐ REPS ☐ REPS ☐ REPS ☐ REPS ☐
☐ BEST INCREASE WEIGHT		
		REPS ☐ REPS ☐ REPS ☐ REPS ☐ REPS ☐
☐ BEST INCREASE WEIGHT		
		REPS ☐ REPS ☐ REPS ☐ REPS ☐ REPS ☐
☐ BEST INCREASE WEIGHT		
		REPS ☐ REPS ☐ REPS ☐ REPS ☐ REPS ☐
☐ BEST INCREASE WEIGHT		
		REPS ☐ REPS ☐ REPS ☐ REPS ☐ REPS ☐
☐ BEST INCREASE WEIGHT		

EXERCISE	SETS	REPS AND DONE!				
		REPS ☐	REPS ☐	REPS ☐	REPS ☐	REPS ☐
[ ] BEST INCREASE — WEIGHT						
		REPS ☐	REPS ☐	REPS ☐	REPS ☐	REPS ☐
[ ] BEST INCREASE — WEIGHT						
		REPS ☐	REPS ☐	REPS ☐	REPS ☐	REPS ☐
[ ] BEST INCREASE — WEIGHT						
		REPS ☐	REPS ☐	REPS ☐	REPS ☐	REPS ☐
[ ] BEST INCREASE — WEIGHT						
		REPS ☐	REPS ☐	REPS ☐	REPS ☐	REPS ☐
[ ] BEST INCREASE — WEIGHT						
		REPS ☐	REPS ☐	REPS ☐	REPS ☐	REPS ☐
[ ] BEST INCREASE — WEIGHT						
		REPS ☐	REPS ☐	REPS ☐	REPS ☐	REPS ☐
[ ] BEST INCREASE — WEIGHT						
		REPS ☐	REPS ☐	REPS ☐	REPS ☐	REPS ☐
[ ] BEST INCREASE — WEIGHT						
		REPS ☐	REPS ☐	REPS ☐	REPS ☐	REPS ☐
[ ] BEST INCREASE — WEIGHT						
		REPS ☐	REPS ☐	REPS ☐	REPS ☐	REPS ☐
[ ] BEST INCREASE — WEIGHT						
		REPS ☐	REPS ☐	REPS ☐	REPS ☐	REPS ☐
[ ] BEST INCREASE — WEIGHT						

EXERCISE	SETS	REPS AND DONE!

		REPS ☐	REPS ☐	REPS ☐	REPS ☐	REPS ☐
☐ BEST INCREASE ◄ WEIGHT ►						
		REPS ☐	REPS ☐	REPS ☐	REPS ☐	REPS ☐
☐ BEST INCREASE ◄ WEIGHT ►						
		REPS ☐	REPS ☐	REPS ☐	REPS ☐	REPS ☐
☐ BEST INCREASE ◄ WEIGHT ►						
		REPS ☐	REPS ☐	REPS ☐	REPS ☐	REPS ☐
☐ BEST INCREASE ◄ WEIGHT ►						
		REPS ☐	REPS ☐	REPS ☐	REPS ☐	REPS ☐
☐ BEST INCREASE ◄ WEIGHT ►						
		REPS ☐	REPS ☐	REPS ☐	REPS ☐	REPS ☐
☐ BEST INCREASE ◄ WEIGHT ►						
		REPS ☐	REPS ☐	REPS ☐	REPS ☐	REPS ☐
☐ BEST INCREASE ◄ WEIGHT ►						
		REPS ☐	REPS ☐	REPS ☐	REPS ☐	REPS ☐
☐ BEST INCREASE ◄ WEIGHT ►						
		REPS ☐	REPS ☐	REPS ☐	REPS ☐	REPS ☐
☐ BEST INCREASE ◄ WEIGHT ►						
		REPS ☐	REPS ☐	REPS ☐	REPS ☐	REPS ☐
☐ BEST INCREASE ◄ WEIGHT ►						

EXERCISE	SETS	REPS AND DONE!				
		✓ REPS ☐	✓ REPS ☐	✓ REPS ☐	✓ REPS ☐	✓ REPS ☐
☐ BEST INCREASE → WEIGHT →		☐	☐	☐	☐	☐
		REPS ☐	REPS ☐	REPS ☐	REPS ☐	REPS ☐
☐ BEST INCREASE → WEIGHT →		☐	☐	☐	☐	☐
		REPS ☐	REPS ☐	REPS ☐	REPS ☐	REPS ☐
☐ BEST INCREASE → WEIGHT →		☐	☐	☐	☐	☐
		REPS ☐	REPS ☐	REPS ☐	REPS ☐	REPS ☐
☐ BEST INCREASE → WEIGHT →		☐	☐	☐	☐	☐
		REPS ☐	REPS ☐	REPS ☐	REPS ☐	REPS ☐
☐ BEST INCREASE → WEIGHT →		☐	☐	☐	☐	☐
		REPS ☐	REPS ☐	REPS ☐	REPS ☐	REPS ☐
☐ BEST INCREASE → WEIGHT →		☐	☐	☐	☐	☐
		REPS ☐	REPS ☐	REPS ☐	REPS ☐	REPS ☐
☐ BEST INCREASE → WEIGHT →		☐	☐	☐	☐	☐
		REPS ☐	REPS ☐	REPS ☐	REPS ☐	REPS ☐
☐ BEST INCREASE → WEIGHT →		☐	☐	☐	☐	☐
		REPS ☐	REPS ☐	REPS ☐	REPS ☐	REPS ☐
☐ BEST INCREASE → WEIGHT →		☐	☐	☐	☐	☐
		REPS ☐	REPS ☐	REPS ☐	REPS ☐	REPS ☐
☐ BEST INCREASE → WEIGHT →		☐	☐	☐	☐	☐
		REPS ☐	REPS ☐	REPS ☐	REPS ☐	REPS ☐
☐ BEST INCREASE → WEIGHT →		☐	☐	☐	☐	☐

EXERCISE	SETS	REPS AND DONE!				
		REPS ☐	REPS ☐	REPS ☐	REPS ☐	REPS ☐
BEST INCREASE → WEIGHT →						
		REPS ☐	REPS ☐	REPS ☐	REPS ☐	REPS ☐
BEST INCREASE → WEIGHT →						
		REPS ☐	REPS ☐	REPS ☐	REPS ☐	REPS ☐
BEST INCREASE → WEIGHT →						
		REPS ☐	REPS ☐	REPS ☐	REPS ☐	REPS ☐
BEST INCREASE → WEIGHT →						
		REPS ☐	REPS ☐	REPS ☐	REPS ☐	REPS ☐
BEST INCREASE → WEIGHT →						
		REPS ☐	REPS ☐	REPS ☐	REPS ☐	REPS ☐
BEST INCREASE → WEIGHT →						
		REPS ☐	REPS ☐	REPS ☐	REPS ☐	REPS ☐
BEST INCREASE → WEIGHT →						
		REPS ☐	REPS ☐	REPS ☐	REPS ☐	REPS ☐
BEST INCREASE → WEIGHT →						
		REPS ☐	REPS ☐	REPS ☐	REPS ☐	REPS ☐
BEST INCREASE → WEIGHT →						
		REPS ☐	REPS ☐	REPS ☐	REPS ☐	REPS ☐
BEST INCREASE → WEIGHT →						
		REPS ☐	REPS ☐	REPS ☐	REPS ☐	REPS ☐
BEST INCREASE → WEIGHT →						

EXERCISE	SETS	REPS AND DONE!				
		REPS ✓	REPS ✓	REPS ✓	REPS ✓	REPS ✓
BEST INCREASE → WEIGHT →						
		REPS	REPS	REPS	REPS	REPS
BEST INCREASE → WEIGHT →						
		REPS	REPS	REPS	REPS	REPS
BEST INCREASE → WEIGHT →						
		REPS	REPS	REPS	REPS	REPS
BEST INCREASE → WEIGHT →						
		REPS	REPS	REPS	REPS	REPS
BEST INCREASE → WEIGHT →						
		REPS	REPS	REPS	REPS	REPS
BEST INCREASE → WEIGHT →						
		REPS	REPS	REPS	REPS	REPS
BEST INCREASE → WEIGHT →						
		REPS	REPS	REPS	REPS	REPS
BEST INCREASE → WEIGHT →						
		REPS	REPS	REPS	REPS	REPS
BEST INCREASE → WEIGHT →						
		REPS	REPS	REPS	REPS	REPS
BEST INCREASE → WEIGHT →						
		REPS	REPS	REPS	REPS	REPS
BEST INCREASE → WEIGHT →						
		REPS	REPS	REPS	REPS	REPS
BEST INCREASE → WEIGHT →						

EXERCISE	SETS	REPS AND DONE!				
		✓	✓	✓	✓	✓
		REPS ☐	REPS ☐	REPS ☐	REPS ☐	REPS ☐
BEST INCREASE — WEIGHT						
		REPS ☐	REPS ☐	REPS ☐	REPS ☐	REPS ☐
BEST INCREASE — WEIGHT						
		REPS ☐	REPS ☐	REPS ☐	REPS ☐	REPS ☐
BEST INCREASE — WEIGHT						
		REPS ☐	REPS ☐	REPS ☐	REPS ☐	REPS ☐
BEST INCREASE — WEIGHT						
		REPS ☐	REPS ☐	REPS ☐	REPS ☐	REPS ☐
BEST INCREASE — WEIGHT						
		REPS ☐	REPS ☐	REPS ☐	REPS ☐	REPS ☐
BEST INCREASE — WEIGHT						
		REPS ☐	REPS ☐	REPS ☐	REPS ☐	REPS ☐
BEST INCREASE — WEIGHT						
		REPS ☐	REPS ☐	REPS ☐	REPS ☐	REPS ☐
BEST INCREASE — WEIGHT						
		REPS ☐	REPS ☐	REPS ☐	REPS ☐	REPS ☐
BEST INCREASE — WEIGHT						
		REPS ☐	REPS ☐	REPS ☐	REPS ☐	REPS ☐
BEST INCREASE — WEIGHT						
		REPS ☐	REPS ☐	REPS ☐	REPS ☐	REPS ☐
BEST INCREASE — WEIGHT						

EXERCISE	SETS	REPS AND DONE!				
		REPS ✓	REPS ✓	REPS ✓	REPS ✓	REPS ✓
BEST INCREASE WEIGHT						
		REPS	REPS	REPS	REPS	REPS
BEST INCREASE WEIGHT						
		REPS	REPS	REPS	REPS	REPS
BEST INCREASE WEIGHT						
		REPS	REPS	REPS	REPS	REPS
BEST INCREASE WEIGHT						
		REPS	REPS	REPS	REPS	REPS
BEST INCREASE WEIGHT						
		REPS	REPS	REPS	REPS	REPS
BEST INCREASE WEIGHT						
		REPS	REPS	REPS	REPS	REPS
BEST INCREASE WEIGHT						
		REPS	REPS	REPS	REPS	REPS
BEST INCREASE WEIGHT						
		REPS	REPS	REPS	REPS	REPS
BEST INCREASE WEIGHT						
		REPS	REPS	REPS	REPS	REPS
BEST INCREASE WEIGHT						
		REPS	REPS	REPS	REPS	REPS
BEST INCREASE WEIGHT						
		REPS	REPS	REPS	REPS	REPS
BEST INCREASE WEIGHT						

EXERCISE	SETS	REPS AND DONE!				
		REPS ☐	REPS ☐	REPS ☐	REPS ☐	REPS ☐
BEST INCREASE ← WEIGHT →						
		REPS ☐	REPS ☐	REPS ☐	REPS ☐	REPS ☐
BEST INCREASE ← WEIGHT →						
		REPS ☐	REPS ☐	REPS ☐	REPS ☐	REPS ☐
BEST INCREASE ← WEIGHT →						
		REPS ☐	REPS ☐	REPS ☐	REPS ☐	REPS ☐
BEST INCREASE ← WEIGHT →						
		REPS ☐	REPS ☐	REPS ☐	REPS ☐	REPS ☐
BEST INCREASE ← WEIGHT →						
		REPS ☐	REPS ☐	REPS ☐	REPS ☐	REPS ☐
BEST INCREASE ← WEIGHT →						
		REPS ☐	REPS ☐	REPS ☐	REPS ☐	REPS ☐
BEST INCREASE ← WEIGHT →						
		REPS ☐	REPS ☐	REPS ☐	REPS ☐	REPS ☐
BEST INCREASE ← WEIGHT →						
		REPS ☐	REPS ☐	REPS ☐	REPS ☐	REPS ☐
BEST INCREASE ← WEIGHT →						

		REPS ✔	REPS ✔	REPS ✔	REPS ✔	REPS ✔
		REPS ☐	REPS ☐	REPS ☐	REPS ☐	REPS ☐
BEST INCREASE ← 🏋 WEIGHT →						
		REPS ☐	REPS ☐	REPS ☐	REPS ☐	REPS ☐
BEST INCREASE ← 🏋 WEIGHT →						
		REPS ☐	REPS ☐	REPS ☐	REPS ☐	REPS ☐
BEST INCREASE ← 🏋 WEIGHT →						
		REPS ☐	REPS ☐	REPS ☐	REPS ☐	REPS ☐
BEST INCREASE ← 🏋 WEIGHT →						
		REPS ☐	REPS ☐	REPS ☐	REPS ☐	REPS ☐
BEST INCREASE ← 🏋 WEIGHT →						
		REPS ☐	REPS ☐	REPS ☐	REPS ☐	REPS ☐
BEST INCREASE ← 🏋 WEIGHT →						
		REPS ☐	REPS ☐	REPS ☐	REPS ☐	REPS ☐
BEST INCREASE ← 🏋 WEIGHT →						
		REPS ☐	REPS ☐	REPS ☐	REPS ☐	REPS ☐
BEST INCREASE ← 🏋 WEIGHT →						
		REPS ☐	REPS ☐	REPS ☐	REPS ☐	REPS ☐
BEST INCREASE ← 🏋 WEIGHT →						
		REPS ☐	REPS ☐	REPS ☐	REPS ☐	REPS ☐
BEST INCREASE ← 🏋 WEIGHT →						
		REPS ☐	REPS ☐	REPS ☐	REPS ☐	REPS ☐
BEST INCREASE ← 🏋 WEIGHT →						

EXERCISE	SETS	REPS AND DONE!				
		REPS ☑	REPS ☑	REPS ☑	REPS ☑	REPS ☑
BEST INCREASE ▸ WEIGHT ▸						
		REPS ☐	REPS ☐	REPS ☐	REPS ☐	REPS ☐
BEST INCREASE ▸ WEIGHT ▸						
		REPS ☐	REPS ☐	REPS ☐	REPS ☐	REPS ☐
BEST INCREASE ▸ WEIGHT ▸						
		REPS ☐	REPS ☐	REPS ☐	REPS ☐	REPS ☐
BEST INCREASE ▸ WEIGHT ▸						
		REPS ☐	REPS ☐	REPS ☐	REPS ☐	REPS ☐
BEST INCREASE ▸ WEIGHT ▸						
		REPS ☐	REPS ☐	REPS ☐	REPS ☐	REPS ☐
BEST INCREASE ▸ WEIGHT ▸						
		REPS ☐	REPS ☐	REPS ☐	REPS ☐	REPS ☐
BEST INCREASE ▸ WEIGHT ▸						
		REPS ☐	REPS ☐	REPS ☐	REPS ☐	REPS ☐
BEST INCREASE ▸ WEIGHT ▸						
		REPS ☐	REPS ☐	REPS ☐	REPS ☐	REPS ☐
BEST INCREASE ▸ WEIGHT ▸						
		REPS ☐	REPS ☐	REPS ☐	REPS ☐	REPS ☐
BEST INCREASE ▸ WEIGHT ▸						
		REPS ☐	REPS ☐	REPS ☐	REPS ☐	REPS ☐
BEST INCREASE ▸ WEIGHT ▸						

EXERCISE	SETS	REPS AND DONE!				
		REPS ☑	REPS ☑	REPS ☑	REPS ☑	REPS ☑
BEST INCREASE → WEIGHT →						
		REPS ☐	REPS ☐	REPS ☐	REPS ☐	REPS ☐
BEST INCREASE → WEIGHT →						
		REPS ☐	REPS ☐	REPS ☐	REPS ☐	REPS ☐
BEST INCREASE → WEIGHT →						
		REPS ☐	REPS ☐	REPS ☐	REPS ☐	REPS ☐
BEST INCREASE → WEIGHT →						
		REPS ☐	REPS ☐	REPS ☐	REPS ☐	REPS ☐
BEST INCREASE → WEIGHT →						
		REPS ☐	REPS ☐	REPS ☐	REPS ☐	REPS ☐
BEST INCREASE → WEIGHT →						
		REPS ☐	REPS ☐	REPS ☐	REPS ☐	REPS ☐
BEST INCREASE → WEIGHT →						
		REPS ☐	REPS ☐	REPS ☐	REPS ☐	REPS ☐
BEST INCREASE → WEIGHT →						
		REPS ☐	REPS ☐	REPS ☐	REPS ☐	REPS ☐
BEST INCREASE → WEIGHT →						
		REPS ☐	REPS ☐	REPS ☐	REPS ☐	REPS ☐
BEST INCREASE → WEIGHT →						
		REPS ☐	REPS ☐	REPS ☐	REPS ☐	REPS ☐
BEST INCREASE → WEIGHT →						

		REPS ☐	REPS ☐	REPS ☐	REPS ☐	REPS ☐
BEST INCREASE WEIGHT						
		REPS ☐	REPS ☐	REPS ☐	REPS ☐	REPS ☐
BEST INCREASE WEIGHT						
		REPS ☐	REPS ☐	REPS ☐	REPS ☐	REPS ☐
BEST INCREASE WEIGHT						
		REPS ☐	REPS ☐	REPS ☐	REPS ☐	REPS ☐
BEST INCREASE WEIGHT						
		REPS ☐	REPS ☐	REPS ☐	REPS ☐	REPS ☐
BEST INCREASE WEIGHT						
		REPS ☐	REPS ☐	REPS ☐	REPS ☐	REPS ☐
BEST INCREASE WEIGHT						
		REPS ☐	REPS ☐	REPS ☐	REPS ☐	REPS ☐
BEST INCREASE WEIGHT						
		REPS ☐	REPS ☐	REPS ☐	REPS ☐	REPS ☐
BEST INCREASE WEIGHT						
		REPS ☐	REPS ☐	REPS ☐	REPS ☐	REPS ☐
BEST INCREASE WEIGHT						
		REPS ☐	REPS ☐	REPS ☐	REPS ☐	REPS ☐
BEST INCREASE WEIGHT						

		REPS ✓	REPS ✓	REPS ✓	REPS ✓	REPS ✓
	BEST INCREASE WEIGHT					
		REPS	REPS	REPS	REPS	REPS
	BEST INCREASE WEIGHT					
		REPS	REPS	REPS	REPS	REPS
	BEST INCREASE WEIGHT					
		REPS	REPS	REPS	REPS	REPS
	BEST INCREASE WEIGHT					
		REPS	REPS	REPS	REPS	REPS
	BEST INCREASE WEIGHT					
		REPS	REPS	REPS	REPS	REPS
	BEST INCREASE WEIGHT					
		REPS	REPS	REPS	REPS	REPS
	BEST INCREASE WEIGHT					
		REPS	REPS	REPS	REPS	REPS
	BEST INCREASE WEIGHT					
		REPS	REPS	REPS	REPS	REPS
	BEST INCREASE WEIGHT					
		REPS	REPS	REPS	REPS	REPS
	BEST INCREASE WEIGHT					
		REPS	REPS	REPS	REPS	REPS
	BEST INCREASE WEIGHT					
		REPS	REPS	REPS	REPS	REPS
	BEST INCREASE WEIGHT					

EXERCISE	SETS	REPS AND DONE!				
		REPS ☐	REPS ☐	REPS ☐	REPS ☐	REPS ☐
BEST INCREASE ← WEIGHT →						
		REPS ☐	REPS ☐	REPS ☐	REPS ☐	REPS ☐
BEST INCREASE ← WEIGHT						
		REPS ☐	REPS ☐	REPS ☐	REPS ☐	REPS ☐
BEST INCREASE ← WEIGHT →						
		REPS ☐	REPS ☐	REPS ☐	REPS ☐	REPS ☐
BEST INCREASE ← WEIGHT →						
		REPS ☐	REPS ☐	REPS ☐	REPS ☐	REPS ☐
BEST INCREASE ← WEIGHT →						
		REPS ☐	REPS ☐	REPS ☐	REPS ☐	REPS ☐
BEST INCREASE ← WEIGHT →						
		REPS ☐	REPS ☐	REPS ☐	REPS ☐	REPS ☐
BEST INCREASE ← WEIGHT →						
		REPS ☐	REPS ☐	REPS ☐	REPS ☐	REPS ☐
BEST INCREASE ← WEIGHT →						
		REPS ☐	REPS ☐	REPS ☐	REPS ☐	REPS ☐
BEST INCREASE ← WEIGHT →						
		REPS ☐	REPS ☐	REPS ☐	REPS ☐	REPS ☐
BEST INCREASE ← WEIGHT →						

EXERCISE	SETS	REPS AND DONE!				
		✔ REPS ☐	✔ REPS ☐	✔ REPS ☐	✔ REPS ☐	✔ REPS ☐
BEST INCREASE WEIGHT	☐					
		REPS ☐	REPS ☐	REPS ☐	REPS ☐	REPS ☐
BEST INCREASE WEIGHT	☐					
		REPS ☐	REPS ☐	REPS ☐	REPS ☐	REPS ☐
BEST INCREASE WEIGHT	☐					
		REPS ☐	REPS ☐	REPS ☐	REPS ☐	REPS ☐
BEST INCREASE WEIGHT	☐					
		REPS ☐	REPS ☐	REPS ☐	REPS ☐	REPS ☐
BEST INCREASE WEIGHT	☐					
		REPS ☐	REPS ☐	REPS ☐	REPS ☐	REPS ☐
BEST INCREASE WEIGHT	☐					
		REPS ☐	REPS ☐	REPS ☐	REPS ☐	REPS ☐
BEST INCREASE WEIGHT	☐					
		REPS ☐	REPS ☐	REPS ☐	REPS ☐	REPS ☐
BEST INCREASE WEIGHT	☐					
		REPS ☐	REPS ☐	REPS ☐	REPS ☐	REPS ☐
BEST INCREASE WEIGHT	☐					
		REPS ☐	REPS ☐	REPS ☐	REPS ☐	REPS ☐
BEST INCREASE WEIGHT	☐					
		REPS ☐	REPS ☐	REPS ☐	REPS ☐	REPS ☐
BEST INCREASE WEIGHT	☐					
		REPS ☐	REPS ☐	REPS ☐	REPS ☐	REPS ☐
BEST INCREASE WEIGHT	☐					

EXERCISE	SETS	REPS ✔	REPS ✔	REPS ✔	REPS ✔	REPS ✔
BEST INCREASE ◄ WEIGHT ►						
		REPS ◯	REPS ◯	REPS ◯	REPS ◯	REPS ◯
BEST INCREASE ◄ WEIGHT ►						
		REPS ◯	REPS ◯	REPS ◯	REPS ◯	REPS ◯
BEST INCREASE ◄ WEIGHT ►						
		REPS ◯	REPS ◯	REPS ◯	REPS ◯	REPS ◯
BEST INCREASE ◄ WEIGHT ►						
		REPS ◯	REPS ◯	REPS ◯	REPS ◯	REPS ◯
BEST INCREASE ◄ WEIGHT ►						
		REPS ◯	REPS ◯	REPS ◯	REPS ◯	REPS ◯
BEST INCREASE ◄ WEIGHT ►						
		REPS ◯	REPS ◯	REPS ◯	REPS ◯	REPS ◯
BEST INCREASE ◄ WEIGHT ►						
		REPS ◯	REPS ◯	REPS ◯	REPS ◯	REPS ◯
BEST INCREASE ◄ WEIGHT ►						
		REPS ◯	REPS ◯	REPS ◯	REPS ◯	REPS ◯
BEST INCREASE ◄ WEIGHT ►						
		REPS ◯	REPS ◯	REPS ◯	REPS ◯	REPS ◯
BEST INCREASE ◄ WEIGHT ►						

EXERCISE	SETS	REPS AND DONE!				
		✔	✔	✔	✔	✔
		REPS ☐	REPS ☐	REPS ☐	REPS ☐	REPS ☐
BEST INCREASE ← WEIGHT →						
		REPS ☐	REPS ☐	REPS ☐	REPS ☐	REPS ☐
BEST INCREASE ← WEIGHT →						
		REPS ☐	REPS ☐	REPS ☐	REPS ☐	REPS ☐
BEST INCREASE ← WEIGHT →						
		REPS ☐	REPS ☐	REPS ☐	REPS ☐	REPS ☐
BEST INCREASE ← WEIGHT →						
		REPS ☐	REPS ☐	REPS ☐	REPS ☐	REPS ☐
BEST INCREASE ← WEIGHT →						
		REPS ☐	REPS ☐	REPS ☐	REPS ☐	REPS ☐
BEST INCREASE ← WEIGHT →						
		REPS ☐	REPS ☐	REPS ☐	REPS ☐	REPS ☐
BEST INCREASE ← WEIGHT →						
		REPS ☐	REPS ☐	REPS ☐	REPS ☐	REPS ☐
BEST INCREASE ← WEIGHT →						
		REPS ☐	REPS ☐	REPS ☐	REPS ☐	REPS ☐
BEST INCREASE ← WEIGHT →						
		REPS ☐	REPS ☐	REPS ☐	REPS ☐	REPS ☐
BEST INCREASE ← WEIGHT →						
		REPS ☐	REPS ☐	REPS ☐	REPS ☐	REPS ☐
BEST INCREASE ← WEIGHT →						
		REPS ☐	REPS ☐	REPS ☐	REPS ☐	REPS ☐
BEST INCREASE ← WEIGHT →						

	SETS	REPS ✓	REPS ✓	REPS ✓	REPS ✓	REPS ✓
	BEST INCREASE ← WEIGHT →					
		REPS	REPS	REPS	REPS	REPS
	BEST INCREASE ← WEIGHT →					
		REPS	REPS	REPS	REPS	REPS
	BEST INCREASE ← WEIGHT →					
		REPS	REPS	REPS	REPS	REPS
	BEST INCREASE ← WEIGHT →					
		REPS	REPS	REPS	REPS	REPS
	BEST INCREASE ← WEIGHT →					
		REPS	REPS	REPS	REPS	REPS
	BEST INCREASE ← WEIGHT →					
		REPS	REPS	REPS	REPS	REPS
	BEST INCREASE ← WEIGHT →					
		REPS	REPS	REPS	REPS	REPS
	BEST INCREASE ← WEIGHT →					
		REPS	REPS	REPS	REPS	REPS
	BEST INCREASE ← WEIGHT →					
		REPS	REPS	REPS	REPS	REPS
	BEST INCREASE ← WEIGHT →					
		REPS	REPS	REPS	REPS	REPS
	BEST INCREASE ← WEIGHT →					

		REPS ✔	REPS ✔	REPS ✔	REPS ✔	REPS ✔
	BEST INCREASE ← WEIGHT →					
		REPS	REPS	REPS	REPS	REPS
	BEST INCREASE ← WEIGHT →					
		REPS	REPS	REPS	REPS	REPS
	BEST INCREASE ← WEIGHT →					
		REPS	REPS	REPS	REPS	REPS
	BEST INCREASE ← WEIGHT →					
		REPS	REPS	REPS	REPS	REPS
	BEST INCREASE ← WEIGHT →					
		REPS	REPS	REPS	REPS	REPS
	BEST INCREASE ← WEIGHT →					
		REPS	REPS	REPS	REPS	REPS
	BEST INCREASE ← WEIGHT →					
		REPS	REPS	REPS	REPS	REPS
	BEST INCREASE ← WEIGHT →					
		REPS	REPS	REPS	REPS	REPS
	BEST INCREASE ← WEIGHT →					
		REPS	REPS	REPS	REPS	REPS
	BEST INCREASE ← WEIGHT →					
		REPS	REPS	REPS	REPS	REPS
	BEST INCREASE ← WEIGHT →					

EXERCISE	SETS	REPS AND DONE!
		REPS ☐ REPS ☐ REPS ☐ REPS ☐ REPS ☐
BEST INCREASE — WEIGHT		
		REPS ☐ REPS ☐ REPS ☐ REPS ☐ REPS ☐
BEST INCREASE — WEIGHT		
		REPS ☐ REPS ☐ REPS ☐ REPS ☐ REPS ☐
BEST INCREASE — WEIGHT		
		REPS ☐ REPS ☐ REPS ☐ REPS ☐ REPS ☐
BEST INCREASE — WEIGHT		
		REPS ☐ REPS ☐ REPS ☐ REPS ☐ REPS ☐
BEST INCREASE — WEIGHT		
		REPS ☐ REPS ☐ REPS ☐ REPS ☐ REPS ☐
BEST INCREASE — WEIGHT		
		REPS ☐ REPS ☐ REPS ☐ REPS ☐ REPS ☐
BEST INCREASE — WEIGHT		
		REPS ☐ REPS ☐ REPS ☐ REPS ☐ REPS ☐
BEST INCREASE — WEIGHT		
		REPS ☐ REPS ☐ REPS ☐ REPS ☐ REPS ☐
BEST INCREASE — WEIGHT		
		REPS ☐ REPS ☐ REPS ☐ REPS ☐ REPS ☐
BEST INCREASE — WEIGHT		
		REPS ☐ REPS ☐ REPS ☐ REPS ☐ REPS ☐
BEST INCREASE — WEIGHT		

EXERCISE — SETS — REPS AND DONE!

	REPS ☐	REPS ☐	REPS ☐	REPS ☐	REPS ☐
BEST INCREASE — WEIGHT					
	REPS ☐	REPS ☐	REPS ☐	REPS ☐	REPS ☐
BEST INCREASE — WEIGHT					
	REPS ☐	REPS ☐	REPS ☐	REPS ☐	REPS ☐
BEST INCREASE — WEIGHT					
	REPS ☐	REPS ☐	REPS ☐	REPS ☐	REPS ☐
BEST INCREASE — WEIGHT					
	REPS ☐	REPS ☐	REPS ☐	REPS ☐	REPS ☐
BEST INCREASE — WEIGHT					
	REPS ☐	REPS ☐	REPS ☐	REPS ☐	REPS ☐
BEST INCREASE — WEIGHT					
	REPS ☐	REPS ☐	REPS ☐	REPS ☐	REPS ☐
BEST INCREASE — WEIGHT					
	REPS ☐	REPS ☐	REPS ☐	REPS ☐	REPS ☐
BEST INCREASE — WEIGHT					
	REPS ☐	REPS ☐	REPS ☐	REPS ☐	REPS ☐
BEST INCREASE — WEIGHT					
	REPS ☐	REPS ☐	REPS ☐	REPS ☐	REPS ☐
BEST INCREASE — WEIGHT					
	REPS ☐	REPS ☐	REPS ☐	REPS ☐	REPS ☐
BEST INCREASE — WEIGHT					
	REPS ☐	REPS ☐	REPS ☐	REPS ☐	REPS ☐
BEST INCREASE — WEIGHT					

EXERCISE	SETS	REPS AND DONE!				
		REPS ☐	REPS ☐	REPS ☐	REPS ☐	REPS ☐
☐ BEST INCREASE → WEIGHT →						
		REPS ☐	REPS ☐	REPS ☐	REPS ☐	REPS ☐
☐ BEST INCREASE → WEIGHT →						
		REPS ☐	REPS ☐	REPS ☐	REPS ☐	REPS ☐
☐ BEST INCREASE → WEIGHT →						
		REPS ☐	REPS ☐	REPS ☐	REPS ☐	REPS ☐
☐ BEST INCREASE → WEIGHT →						
		REPS ☐	REPS ☐	REPS ☐	REPS ☐	REPS ☐
☐ BEST INCREASE → WEIGHT →						
		REPS ☐	REPS ☐	REPS ☐	REPS ☐	REPS ☐
☐ BEST INCREASE → WEIGHT →						
		REPS ☐	REPS ☐	REPS ☐	REPS ☐	REPS ☐
☐ BEST INCREASE → WEIGHT →						
		REPS ☐	REPS ☐	REPS ☐	REPS ☐	REPS ☐
☐ BEST INCREASE → WEIGHT →						
		REPS ☐	REPS ☐	REPS ☐	REPS ☐	REPS ☐
☐ BEST INCREASE → WEIGHT →						
		REPS ☐	REPS ☐	REPS ☐	REPS ☐	REPS ☐
☐ BEST INCREASE → WEIGHT →						

EXERCISE	SETS	REPS AND DONE!				
		REPS ✓	REPS ✓	REPS ✓	REPS ✓	REPS ✓
BEST INCREASE — WEIGHT						
		REPS	REPS	REPS	REPS	REPS
BEST INCREASE — WEIGHT						
		REPS	REPS	REPS	REPS	REPS
BEST INCREASE — WEIGHT						
		REPS	REPS	REPS	REPS	REPS
BEST INCREASE — WEIGHT						
		REPS	REPS	REPS	REPS	REPS
BEST INCREASE — WEIGHT						
		REPS	REPS	REPS	REPS	REPS
BEST INCREASE — WEIGHT						
		REPS	REPS	REPS	REPS	REPS
BEST INCREASE — WEIGHT						
		REPS	REPS	REPS	REPS	REPS
BEST INCREASE — WEIGHT						
		REPS	REPS	REPS	REPS	REPS
BEST INCREASE — WEIGHT						
		REPS	REPS	REPS	REPS	REPS
BEST INCREASE — WEIGHT						
		REPS	REPS	REPS	REPS	REPS
BEST INCREASE — WEIGHT						

EXERCISE — SETS — REPS AND DONE!

EXERCISE	SETS	REPS ✔	REPS ✔	REPS ✔	REPS ✔	REPS ✔
BEST INCREASE — WEIGHT						
		REPS	REPS	REPS	REPS	REPS
BEST INCREASE — WEIGHT						
		REPS	REPS	REPS	REPS	REPS
BEST INCREASE — WEIGHT						
		REPS	REPS	REPS	REPS	REPS
BEST INCREASE — WEIGHT						
		REPS	REPS	REPS	REPS	REPS
BEST INCREASE — WEIGHT						
		REPS	REPS	REPS	REPS	REPS
BEST INCREASE — WEIGHT						
		REPS	REPS	REPS	REPS	REPS
BEST INCREASE — WEIGHT						
		REPS	REPS	REPS	REPS	REPS
BEST INCREASE — WEIGHT						
		REPS	REPS	REPS	REPS	REPS
BEST INCREASE — WEIGHT						
		REPS	REPS	REPS	REPS	REPS
BEST INCREASE — WEIGHT						

EXERCISE	SETS	REPS AND DONE!

		REPS ✓	REPS ✓	REPS ✓	REPS ✓	REPS ✓
BEST INCREASE — WEIGHT						
		REPS	REPS	REPS	REPS	REPS
BEST INCREASE — WEIGHT						
		REPS	REPS	REPS	REPS	REPS
BEST INCREASE — WEIGHT						
		REPS	REPS	REPS	REPS	REPS
BEST INCREASE — WEIGHT						
		REPS	REPS	REPS	REPS	REPS
BEST INCREASE — WEIGHT						
		REPS	REPS	REPS	REPS	REPS
BEST INCREASE — WEIGHT						
		REPS	REPS	REPS	REPS	REPS
BEST INCREASE — WEIGHT						
		REPS	REPS	REPS	REPS	REPS
BEST INCREASE — WEIGHT						
		REPS	REPS	REPS	REPS	REPS
BEST INCREASE — WEIGHT						
		REPS	REPS	REPS	REPS	REPS
BEST INCREASE — WEIGHT						
		REPS	REPS	REPS	REPS	REPS
BEST INCREASE — WEIGHT						
		REPS	REPS	REPS	REPS	REPS
BEST INCREASE — WEIGHT						

EXERCISE	SETS	REPS ✓	REPS ✓	REPS ✓	REPS ✓	REPS ✓
BEST INCREASE ◄ WEIGHT ►						
		REPS	REPS	REPS	REPS	REPS
BEST INCREASE ◄ WEIGHT ►						
		REPS	REPS	REPS	REPS	REPS
BEST INCREASE ◄ WEIGHT ►						
		REPS	REPS	REPS	REPS	REPS
BEST INCREASE ◄ WEIGHT ►						
		REPS	REPS	REPS	REPS	REPS
BEST INCREASE ◄ WEIGHT ►						
		REPS	REPS	REPS	REPS	REPS
BEST INCREASE ◄ WEIGHT ►						
		REPS	REPS	REPS	REPS	REPS
BEST INCREASE ◄ WEIGHT ►						
		REPS	REPS	REPS	REPS	REPS
BEST INCREASE ◄ WEIGHT ►						
		REPS	REPS	REPS	REPS	REPS
BEST INCREASE ◄ WEIGHT ►						
		REPS	REPS	REPS	REPS	REPS
BEST INCREASE ◄ WEIGHT ►						
		REPS	REPS	REPS	REPS	REPS
BEST INCREASE ◄ WEIGHT ►						

●——EXERCISE———●	SETS ●——	REPS AND DONE! ——●

EXERCISE	BEST INCREASE ◄ WEIGHT ►	REPS ✓	REPS ✓	REPS ✓	REPS ✓	REPS ✓
	BEST INCREASE ◄ WEIGHT ►					
		REPS	REPS	REPS	REPS	REPS
	BEST INCREASE ◄ WEIGHT ►					
		REPS	REPS	REPS	REPS	REPS
	BEST INCREASE ◄ WEIGHT ►					
		REPS	REPS	REPS	REPS	REPS
	BEST INCREASE ◄ WEIGHT ►					
		REPS	REPS	REPS	REPS	REPS
	BEST INCREASE ◄ WEIGHT ►					
		REPS	REPS	REPS	REPS	REPS
	BEST INCREASE ◄ WEIGHT ►					
		REPS	REPS	REPS	REPS	REPS
	BEST INCREASE ◄ WEIGHT ►					
		REPS	REPS	REPS	REPS	REPS
	BEST INCREASE ◄ WEIGHT ►					
		REPS	REPS	REPS	REPS	REPS
	BEST INCREASE ◄ WEIGHT ►					
		REPS	REPS	REPS	REPS	REPS
	BEST INCREASE ◄ WEIGHT ►					
		REPS	REPS	REPS	REPS	REPS
	BEST INCREASE ◄ WEIGHT ►					
		REPS	REPS	REPS	REPS	REPS
	BEST INCREASE ◄ WEIGHT ►					

EXERCISE	SETS	REPS ✓	REPS ✓	REPS ✓	REPS ✓	REPS ✓
BEST INCREASE — WEIGHT						
		REPS	REPS	REPS	REPS	REPS
BEST INCREASE — WEIGHT						
		REPS	REPS	REPS	REPS	REPS
BEST INCREASE — WEIGHT						
		REPS	REPS	REPS	REPS	REPS
BEST INCREASE — WEIGHT						
		REPS	REPS	REPS	REPS	REPS
BEST INCREASE — WEIGHT						
		REPS	REPS	REPS	REPS	REPS
BEST INCREASE — WEIGHT						
		REPS	REPS	REPS	REPS	REPS
BEST INCREASE — WEIGHT						
		REPS	REPS	REPS	REPS	REPS
BEST INCREASE — WEIGHT						
		REPS	REPS	REPS	REPS	REPS
BEST INCREASE — WEIGHT						
		REPS	REPS	REPS	REPS	REPS
BEST INCREASE — WEIGHT						

EXERCISE	SETS	REPS AND DONE!				
		REPS ✓	REPS ✓	REPS ✓	REPS ✓	REPS ✓
BEST INCREASE WEIGHT						
		REPS	REPS	REPS	REPS	REPS
BEST INCREASE WEIGHT						
		REPS	REPS	REPS	REPS	REPS
BEST INCREASE WEIGHT						
		REPS	REPS	REPS	REPS	REPS
BEST INCREASE WEIGHT						
		REPS	REPS	REPS	REPS	REPS
BEST INCREASE WEIGHT						
		REPS	REPS	REPS	REPS	REPS
BEST INCREASE WEIGHT						
		REPS	REPS	REPS	REPS	REPS
BEST INCREASE WEIGHT						
		REPS	REPS	REPS	REPS	REPS
BEST INCREASE WEIGHT						
		REPS	REPS	REPS	REPS	REPS
BEST INCREASE WEIGHT						
		REPS	REPS	REPS	REPS	REPS
BEST INCREASE WEIGHT						
		REPS	REPS	REPS	REPS	REPS
BEST INCREASE WEIGHT						

EXERCISE	SETS	REPS AND DONE!

EXERCISE		REPS ✓	REPS ✓	REPS ✓	REPS ✓	REPS ✓
	BEST INCREASE — WEIGHT					
		REPS	REPS	REPS	REPS	REPS
	BEST INCREASE — WEIGHT					
		REPS	REPS	REPS	REPS	REPS
	BEST INCREASE — WEIGHT					
		REPS	REPS	REPS	REPS	REPS
	BEST INCREASE — WEIGHT					
		REPS	REPS	REPS	REPS	REPS
	BEST INCREASE — WEIGHT					
		REPS	REPS	REPS	REPS	REPS
	BEST INCREASE — WEIGHT					
		REPS	REPS	REPS	REPS	REPS
	BEST INCREASE — WEIGHT					
		REPS	REPS	REPS	REPS	REPS
	BEST INCREASE — WEIGHT					
		REPS	REPS	REPS	REPS	REPS
	BEST INCREASE — WEIGHT					
		REPS	REPS	REPS	REPS	REPS
	BEST INCREASE — WEIGHT					
		REPS	REPS	REPS	REPS	REPS
	BEST INCREASE — WEIGHT					
		REPS	REPS	REPS	REPS	REPS
	BEST INCREASE — WEIGHT					

EXERCISE •——————• SETS •————— REPS AND DONE! ——————•

EXERCISE	SETS	REPS ✔	REPS ✔	REPS ✔	REPS ✔	REPS ✔
BEST INCREASE → WEIGHT →						
BEST INCREASE → WEIGHT →		REPS	REPS	REPS	REPS	REPS
BEST INCREASE → WEIGHT →		REPS	REPS	REPS	REPS	REPS
BEST INCREASE → WEIGHT →		REPS	REPS	REPS	REPS	REPS
BEST INCREASE → WEIGHT →		REPS	REPS	REPS	REPS	REPS
BEST INCREASE → WEIGHT →		REPS	REPS	REPS	REPS	REPS
BEST INCREASE → WEIGHT →		REPS	REPS	REPS	REPS	REPS
BEST INCREASE → WEIGHT →		REPS	REPS	REPS	REPS	REPS
BEST INCREASE → WEIGHT →		REPS	REPS	REPS	REPS	REPS
BEST INCREASE → WEIGHT →		REPS	REPS	REPS	REPS	REPS
BEST INCREASE → WEIGHT →		REPS	REPS	REPS	REPS	REPS
BEST INCREASE → WEIGHT →		REPS	REPS	REPS	REPS	REPS

EXERCISE	SETS	REPS ✓	REPS ✓	REPS ✓	REPS ✓	REPS ✓
BEST INCREASE ← WEIGHT						
		REPS ☐	REPS ☐	REPS ☐	REPS ☐	REPS ☐
BEST INCREASE ← WEIGHT						
		REPS ☐	REPS ☐	REPS ☐	REPS ☐	REPS ☐
BEST INCREASE ← WEIGHT						
		REPS ☐	REPS ☐	REPS ☐	REPS ☐	REPS ☐
BEST INCREASE ← WEIGHT						
		REPS ☐	REPS ☐	REPS ☐	REPS ☐	REPS ☐
BEST INCREASE ← WEIGHT						
		REPS ☐	REPS ☐	REPS ☐	REPS ☐	REPS ☐
BEST INCREASE ← WEIGHT						
		REPS ☐	REPS ☐	REPS ☐	REPS ☐	REPS ☐
BEST INCREASE ← WEIGHT						
		REPS ☐	REPS ☐	REPS ☐	REPS ☐	REPS ☐
BEST INCREASE ← WEIGHT						
		REPS ☐	REPS ☐	REPS ☐	REPS ☐	REPS ☐
BEST INCREASE ← WEIGHT						
		REPS ☐	REPS ☐	REPS ☐	REPS ☐	REPS ☐
BEST INCREASE ← WEIGHT						
		REPS ☐	REPS ☐	REPS ☐	REPS ☐	REPS ☐
BEST INCREASE ← WEIGHT						
		REPS ☐	REPS ☐	REPS ☐	REPS ☐	REPS ☐
BEST INCREASE ← WEIGHT						

EXERCISE	SETS	REPS AND DONE!				
		REPS ☐	REPS ☐	REPS ☐	REPS ☐	REPS ☐
BEST INCREASE → WEIGHT →						
		REPS ☐	REPS ☐	REPS ☐	REPS ☐	REPS ☐
BEST INCREASE → WEIGHT →						
		REPS ☐	REPS ☐	REPS ☐	REPS ☐	REPS ☐
BEST INCREASE → WEIGHT →						
		REPS ☐	REPS ☐	REPS ☐	REPS ☐	REPS ☐
BEST INCREASE → WEIGHT →						
		REPS ☐	REPS ☐	REPS ☐	REPS ☐	REPS ☐
BEST INCREASE → WEIGHT →						
		REPS ☐	REPS ☐	REPS ☐	REPS ☐	REPS ☐
BEST INCREASE → WEIGHT →						
		REPS ☐	REPS ☐	REPS ☐	REPS ☐	REPS ☐
BEST INCREASE → WEIGHT →						
		REPS ☐	REPS ☐	REPS ☐	REPS ☐	REPS ☐
BEST INCREASE → WEIGHT →						
		REPS ☐	REPS ☐	REPS ☐	REPS ☐	REPS ☐
BEST INCREASE → WEIGHT →						
		REPS ☐	REPS ☐	REPS ☐	REPS ☐	REPS ☐
BEST INCREASE → WEIGHT →						
		REPS ☐	REPS ☐	REPS ☐	REPS ☐	REPS ☐
BEST INCREASE → WEIGHT →						

EXERCISE	SETS	REPS AND DONE!				
		REPS ☐	REPS ☐	REPS ☐	REPS ☐	REPS ☐
	BEST INCREASE WEIGHT					
		REPS ☐	REPS ☐	REPS ☐	REPS ☐	REPS ☐
	BEST INCREASE WEIGHT					
		REPS ☐	REPS ☐	REPS ☐	REPS ☐	REPS ☐
	BEST INCREASE WEIGHT					
		REPS ☐	REPS ☐	REPS ☐	REPS ☐	REPS ☐
	BEST INCREASE WEIGHT					
		REPS ☐	REPS ☐	REPS ☐	REPS ☐	REPS ☐
	BEST INCREASE WEIGHT					
		REPS ☐	REPS ☐	REPS ☐	REPS ☐	REPS ☐
	BEST INCREASE WEIGHT					
		REPS ☐	REPS ☐	REPS ☐	REPS ☐	REPS ☐
	BEST INCREASE WEIGHT					
		REPS ☐	REPS ☐	REPS ☐	REPS ☐	REPS ☐
	BEST INCREASE WEIGHT					
		REPS ☐	REPS ☐	REPS ☐	REPS ☐	REPS ☐
	BEST INCREASE WEIGHT					
		REPS ☐	REPS ☐	REPS ☐	REPS ☐	REPS ☐
	BEST INCREASE WEIGHT					

		REPS ☐	REPS ☐	REPS ☐	REPS ☐	REPS ☐
BEST INCREASE ◄ WEIGHT ►						
		REPS ☐	REPS ☐	REPS ☐	REPS ☐	REPS ☐
BEST INCREASE ◄ WEIGHT ►						
		REPS ☐	REPS ☐	REPS ☐	REPS ☐	REPS ☐
BEST INCREASE ◄ WEIGHT ►						
		REPS ☐	REPS ☐	REPS ☐	REPS ☐	REPS ☐
BEST INCREASE ◄ WEIGHT ►						
		REPS ☐	REPS ☐	REPS ☐	REPS ☐	REPS ☐
BEST INCREASE ◄ WEIGHT ►						
		REPS ☐	REPS ☐	REPS ☐	REPS ☐	REPS ☐
BEST INCREASE ◄ WEIGHT ►						
		REPS ☐	REPS ☐	REPS ☐	REPS ☐	REPS ☐
BEST INCREASE ◄ WEIGHT ►						
		REPS ☐	REPS ☐	REPS ☐	REPS ☐	REPS ☐
BEST INCREASE ◄ WEIGHT ►						
		REPS ☐	REPS ☐	REPS ☐	REPS ☐	REPS ☐
BEST INCREASE ◄ WEIGHT ►						
		REPS ☐	REPS ☐	REPS ☐	REPS ☐	REPS ☐
BEST INCREASE ◄ WEIGHT ►						
		REPS ☐	REPS ☐	REPS ☐	REPS ☐	REPS ☐
BEST INCREASE ◄ WEIGHT ►						

EXERCISE • SETS • REPS AND DONE!

EXERCISE	SETS	REPS ✓	REPS ✓	REPS ✓	REPS ✓	REPS ✓
BEST INCREASE — WEIGHT						
		REPS	REPS	REPS	REPS	REPS
BEST INCREASE — WEIGHT						
		REPS	REPS	REPS	REPS	REPS
BEST INCREASE — WEIGHT						
		REPS	REPS	REPS	REPS	REPS
BEST INCREASE — WEIGHT						
		REPS	REPS	REPS	REPS	REPS
BEST INCREASE — WEIGHT						
		REPS	REPS	REPS	REPS	REPS
BEST INCREASE — WEIGHT						
		REPS	REPS	REPS	REPS	REPS
BEST INCREASE — WEIGHT						
		REPS	REPS	REPS	REPS	REPS
BEST INCREASE — WEIGHT						
		REPS	REPS	REPS	REPS	REPS
BEST INCREASE — WEIGHT						
		REPS	REPS	REPS	REPS	REPS
BEST INCREASE — WEIGHT						
		REPS	REPS	REPS	REPS	REPS
BEST INCREASE — WEIGHT						

EXERCISE	SETS	REPS AND DONE!				
		REPS ✓	REPS ✓	REPS ✓	REPS ✓	REPS ✓
BEST INCREASE — WEIGHT						
		REPS	REPS	REPS	REPS	REPS
BEST INCREASE — WEIGHT						
		REPS	REPS	REPS	REPS	REPS
BEST INCREASE — WEIGHT						
		REPS	REPS	REPS	REPS	REPS
BEST INCREASE — WEIGHT						
		REPS	REPS	REPS	REPS	REPS
BEST INCREASE — WEIGHT						
		REPS	REPS	REPS	REPS	REPS
BEST INCREASE — WEIGHT						
		REPS	REPS	REPS	REPS	REPS
BEST INCREASE — WEIGHT						
		REPS	REPS	REPS	REPS	REPS
BEST INCREASE — WEIGHT						
		REPS	REPS	REPS	REPS	REPS
BEST INCREASE — WEIGHT						
		REPS	REPS	REPS	REPS	REPS
BEST INCREASE — WEIGHT						
		REPS	REPS	REPS	REPS	REPS
BEST INCREASE — WEIGHT						

EXERCISE	SETS	REPS ✔	REPS ✔	REPS ✔	REPS ✔	REPS ✔
BEST INCREASE — WEIGHT						
		REPS ☐	REPS ☐	REPS ☐	REPS ☐	REPS ☐
BEST INCREASE — WEIGHT						
		REPS ☐	REPS ☐	REPS ☐	REPS ☐	REPS ☐
BEST INCREASE — WEIGHT						
		REPS ☐	REPS ☐	REPS ☐	REPS ☐	REPS ☐
BEST INCREASE — WEIGHT						
		REPS ☐	REPS ☐	REPS ☐	REPS ☐	REPS ☐
BEST INCREASE — WEIGHT						
		REPS ☐	REPS ☐	REPS ☐	REPS ☐	REPS ☐
BEST INCREASE — WEIGHT						
		REPS ☐	REPS ☐	REPS ☐	REPS ☐	REPS ☐
BEST INCREASE — WEIGHT						
		REPS ☐	REPS ☐	REPS ☐	REPS ☐	REPS ☐
BEST INCREASE — WEIGHT						
		REPS ☐	REPS ☐	REPS ☐	REPS ☐	REPS ☐
BEST INCREASE — WEIGHT						
		REPS ☐	REPS ☐	REPS ☐	REPS ☐	REPS ☐
BEST INCREASE — WEIGHT						
		REPS ☐	REPS ☐	REPS ☐	REPS ☐	REPS ☐
BEST INCREASE — WEIGHT						

EXERCISE	SETS	REPS AND DONE!				
		REPS ✓	REPS ✓	REPS ✓	REPS ✓	REPS ✓
BEST INCREASE ← WEIGHT						
		REPS	REPS	REPS	REPS	REPS
BEST INCREASE ← WEIGHT						
		REPS	REPS	REPS	REPS	REPS
BEST INCREASE ← WEIGHT						
		REPS	REPS	REPS	REPS	REPS
BEST INCREASE ← WEIGHT						
		REPS	REPS	REPS	REPS	REPS
BEST INCREASE ← WEIGHT						
		REPS	REPS	REPS	REPS	REPS
BEST INCREASE ← WEIGHT						
		REPS	REPS	REPS	REPS	REPS
BEST INCREASE ← WEIGHT						
		REPS	REPS	REPS	REPS	REPS
BEST INCREASE ← WEIGHT						
		REPS	REPS	REPS	REPS	REPS
BEST INCREASE ← WEIGHT						
		REPS	REPS	REPS	REPS	REPS
BEST INCREASE ← WEIGHT						
		REPS	REPS	REPS	REPS	REPS
BEST INCREASE ← WEIGHT						
		REPS	REPS	REPS	REPS	REPS
BEST INCREASE ← WEIGHT						

		REPS ☐	REPS ☐	REPS ☐	REPS ☐	REPS ☐
BEST INCREASE ◄ 🏋 WEIGHT ►						
		REPS ☐	REPS ☐	REPS ☐	REPS ☐	REPS ☐
BEST INCREASE ◄ 🏋 WEIGHT ►						
		REPS ☐	REPS ☐	REPS ☐	REPS ☐	REPS ☐
BEST INCREASE ◄ 🏋 WEIGHT ►						
		REPS ☐	REPS ☐	REPS ☐	REPS ☐	REPS ☐
BEST INCREASE ◄ 🏋 WEIGHT ►						
		REPS ☐	REPS ☐	REPS ☐	REPS ☐	REPS ☐
BEST INCREASE ◄ 🏋 WEIGHT ►						
		REPS ☐	REPS ☐	REPS ☐	REPS ☐	REPS ☐
BEST INCREASE ◄ 🏋 WEIGHT ►						
		REPS ☐	REPS ☐	REPS ☐	REPS ☐	REPS ☐
BEST INCREASE ◄ 🏋 WEIGHT ►						
		REPS ☐	REPS ☐	REPS ☐	REPS ☐	REPS ☐
BEST INCREASE ◄ 🏋 WEIGHT ►						
		REPS ☐	REPS ☐	REPS ☐	REPS ☐	REPS ☐
BEST INCREASE ◄ 🏋 WEIGHT ►						

EXERCISE   •   SETS   •   REPS AND DONE!   •

	REPS ✓	REPS ✓	REPS ✓	REPS ✓	REPS ✓
BEST INCREASE — WEIGHT					
	REPS	REPS	REPS	REPS	REPS
BEST INCREASE — WEIGHT					
	REPS	REPS	REPS	REPS	REPS
BEST INCREASE — WEIGHT					
	REPS	REPS	REPS	REPS	REPS
BEST INCREASE — WEIGHT					
	REPS	REPS	REPS	REPS	REPS
BEST INCREASE — WEIGHT					
	REPS	REPS	REPS	REPS	REPS
BEST INCREASE — WEIGHT					
	REPS	REPS	REPS	REPS	REPS
BEST INCREASE — WEIGHT					
	REPS	REPS	REPS	REPS	REPS
BEST INCREASE — WEIGHT					
	REPS	REPS	REPS	REPS	REPS
BEST INCREASE — WEIGHT					
	REPS	REPS	REPS	REPS	REPS
BEST INCREASE — WEIGHT					

EXERCISE	SETS	REPS ✓	REPS ✓	REPS ✓	REPS ✓	REPS ✓
BEST INCREASE ← WEIGHT →						
		REPS ⬭	REPS ⬭	REPS ⬭	REPS ⬭	REPS ⬭
BEST INCREASE ← WEIGHT →						
		REPS ⬭	REPS ⬭	REPS ⬭	REPS ⬭	REPS ⬭
BEST INCREASE ← WEIGHT →						
		REPS ⬭	REPS ⬭	REPS ⬭	REPS ⬭	REPS ⬭
BEST INCREASE ← WEIGHT →						
		REPS ⬭	REPS ⬭	REPS ⬭	REPS ⬭	REPS ⬭
BEST INCREASE ← WEIGHT →						
		REPS ⬭	REPS ⬭	REPS ⬭	REPS ⬭	REPS ⬭
BEST INCREASE ← WEIGHT →						
		REPS ⬭	REPS ⬭	REPS ⬭	REPS ⬭	REPS ⬭
BEST INCREASE ← WEIGHT →						
		REPS ⬭	REPS ⬭	REPS ⬭	REPS ⬭	REPS ⬭
BEST INCREASE ← WEIGHT →						
		REPS ⬭	REPS ⬭	REPS ⬭	REPS ⬭	REPS ⬭
BEST INCREASE ← WEIGHT →						
		REPS ⬭	REPS ⬭	REPS ⬭	REPS ⬭	REPS ⬭
BEST INCREASE ← WEIGHT →						
		REPS ⬭	REPS ⬭	REPS ⬭	REPS ⬭	REPS ⬭
BEST INCREASE ← WEIGHT →						

EXERCISE	SETS	REPS AND DONE!

		REPS ✓	REPS ✓	REPS ✓	REPS ✓	REPS ✓

BEST INCREASE — WEIGHT

| | | REPS | REPS | REPS | REPS | REPS |

BEST INCREASE — WEIGHT

| | | REPS | REPS | REPS | REPS | REPS |

BEST INCREASE — WEIGHT

| | | REPS | REPS | REPS | REPS | REPS |

BEST INCREASE — WEIGHT

| | | REPS | REPS | REPS | REPS | REPS |

BEST INCREASE — WEIGHT

| | | REPS | REPS | REPS | REPS | REPS |

BEST INCREASE — WEIGHT

| | | REPS | REPS | REPS | REPS | REPS |

BEST INCREASE — WEIGHT

| | | REPS | REPS | REPS | REPS | REPS |

BEST INCREASE — WEIGHT

| | | REPS | REPS | REPS | REPS | REPS |

BEST INCREASE — WEIGHT

| | | REPS | REPS | REPS | REPS | REPS |

BEST INCREASE — WEIGHT

| | | REPS | REPS | REPS | REPS | REPS |

BEST INCREASE — WEIGHT

| | | REPS | REPS | REPS | REPS | REPS |

BEST INCREASE — WEIGHT

EXERCISE	SETS	REPS AND DONE!				
		REPS ☐	REPS ☐	REPS ☐	REPS ☐	REPS ☐
BEST INCREASE → WEIGHT →						
		REPS ☐	REPS ☐	REPS ☐	REPS ☐	REPS ☐
BEST INCREASE → WEIGHT →						
		REPS ☐	REPS ☐	REPS ☐	REPS ☐	REPS ☐
BEST INCREASE → WEIGHT →						
		REPS ☐	REPS ☐	REPS ☐	REPS ☐	REPS ☐
BEST INCREASE → WEIGHT →						
		REPS ☐	REPS ☐	REPS ☐	REPS ☐	REPS ☐
BEST INCREASE → WEIGHT →						
		REPS ☐	REPS ☐	REPS ☐	REPS ☐	REPS ☐
BEST INCREASE → WEIGHT →						
		REPS ☐	REPS ☐	REPS ☐	REPS ☐	REPS ☐
BEST INCREASE → WEIGHT →						
		REPS ☐	REPS ☐	REPS ☐	REPS ☐	REPS ☐
BEST INCREASE → WEIGHT →						
		REPS ☐	REPS ☐	REPS ☐	REPS ☐	REPS ☐
BEST INCREASE → WEIGHT →						
		REPS ☐	REPS ☐	REPS ☐	REPS ☐	REPS ☐
BEST INCREASE → WEIGHT →						
		REPS ☐	REPS ☐	REPS ☐	REPS ☐	REPS ☐
BEST INCREASE → WEIGHT →						

EXERCISE	SETS	REPS AND DONE!

	REPS ✓	REPS ✓	REPS ✓	REPS ✓	REPS ✓
BEST INCREASE ← WEIGHT →					
	REPS	REPS	REPS	REPS	REPS
BEST INCREASE ← WEIGHT →					
	REPS	REPS	REPS	REPS	REPS
BEST INCREASE ← WEIGHT →					
	REPS	REPS	REPS	REPS	REPS
BEST INCREASE ← WEIGHT →					
	REPS	REPS	REPS	REPS	REPS
BEST INCREASE ← WEIGHT →					
	REPS	REPS	REPS	REPS	REPS
BEST INCREASE ← WEIGHT →					
	REPS	REPS	REPS	REPS	REPS
BEST INCREASE ← WEIGHT →					
	REPS	REPS	REPS	REPS	REPS
BEST INCREASE ← WEIGHT →					
	REPS	REPS	REPS	REPS	REPS
BEST INCREASE ← WEIGHT →					
	REPS	REPS	REPS	REPS	REPS
BEST INCREASE ← WEIGHT →					
	REPS	REPS	REPS	REPS	REPS
BEST INCREASE ← WEIGHT →					
	REPS	REPS	REPS	REPS	REPS
BEST INCREASE ← WEIGHT →					

	REPS ✓	REPS ✓	REPS ✓	REPS ✓	REPS ✓
BEST INCREASE ← WEIGHT →					
	REPS ⬭	REPS ⬭	REPS ⬭	REPS ⬭	REPS ⬭
BEST INCREASE ← WEIGHT →					
	REPS ⬭	REPS ⬭	REPS ⬭	REPS ⬭	REPS ⬭
BEST INCREASE ← WEIGHT →					
	REPS ⬭	REPS ⬭	REPS ⬭	REPS ⬭	REPS ⬭
BEST INCREASE ← WEIGHT →					
	REPS ⬭	REPS ⬭	REPS ⬭	REPS ⬭	REPS ⬭
BEST INCREASE ← WEIGHT →					
	REPS ⬭	REPS ⬭	REPS ⬭	REPS ⬭	REPS ⬭
BEST INCREASE ← WEIGHT →					
	REPS ⬭	REPS ⬭	REPS ⬭	REPS ⬭	REPS ⬭
BEST INCREASE ← WEIGHT →					
	REPS ⬭	REPS ⬭	REPS ⬭	REPS ⬭	REPS ⬭
BEST INCREASE ← WEIGHT →					
	REPS ⬭	REPS ⬭	REPS ⬭	REPS ⬭	REPS ⬭
BEST INCREASE ← WEIGHT →					
	REPS ⬭	REPS ⬭	REPS ⬭	REPS ⬭	REPS ⬭
BEST INCREASE ← WEIGHT →					
	REPS ⬭	REPS ⬭	REPS ⬭	REPS ⬭	REPS ⬭
BEST INCREASE ← WEIGHT →					
	REPS ⬭	REPS ⬭	REPS ⬭	REPS ⬭	REPS ⬭
BEST INCREASE ← WEIGHT →					

EXERCISE	SETS	✓	✓	✓	✓	✓
		REPS ☐	REPS ☐	REPS ☐	REPS ☐	REPS ☐
☐ BEST INCREASE ◄ WEIGHT ►						
		REPS ☐	REPS ☐	REPS ☐	REPS ☐	REPS ☐
☐ BEST INCREASE ◄ WEIGHT ►						
		REPS ☐	REPS ☐	REPS ☐	REPS ☐	REPS ☐
☐ BEST INCREASE ◄ WEIGHT ►						
		REPS ☐	REPS ☐	REPS ☐	REPS ☐	REPS ☐
☐ BEST INCREASE ◄ WEIGHT ►						
		REPS ☐	REPS ☐	REPS ☐	REPS ☐	REPS ☐
☐ BEST INCREASE ◄ WEIGHT ►						
		REPS ☐	REPS ☐	REPS ☐	REPS ☐	REPS ☐
☐ BEST INCREASE ◄ WEIGHT ►						
		REPS ☐	REPS ☐	REPS ☐	REPS ☐	REPS ☐
☐ BEST INCREASE ◄ WEIGHT ►						
		REPS ☐	REPS ☐	REPS ☐	REPS ☐	REPS ☐
☐ BEST INCREASE ◄ WEIGHT ►						
		REPS ☐	REPS ☐	REPS ☐	REPS ☐	REPS ☐
☐ BEST INCREASE ◄ WEIGHT ►						
		REPS ☐	REPS ☐	REPS ☐	REPS ☐	REPS ☐
☐ BEST INCREASE ◄ WEIGHT ►						
		REPS ☐	REPS ☐	REPS ☐	REPS ☐	REPS ☐
☐ BEST INCREASE ◄ WEIGHT ►						

EXERCISE ● SETS ● REPS AND DONE! ●

		✓	✓	✓	✓	✓
		REPS ◯	REPS ◯	REPS ◯	REPS ◯	REPS ◯
BEST INCREASE ◀ WEIGHT ▶						
		REPS ◯	REPS ◯	REPS ◯	REPS ◯	REPS ◯
BEST INCREASE ◀ WEIGHT ▶						
		REPS ◯	REPS ◯	REPS ◯	REPS ◯	REPS ◯
BEST INCREASE ◀ WEIGHT ▶						
		REPS ◯	REPS ◯	REPS ◯	REPS ◯	REPS ◯
BEST INCREASE ◀ WEIGHT ▶						
		REPS ◯	REPS ◯	REPS ◯	REPS ◯	REPS ◯
BEST INCREASE ◀ WEIGHT ▶						
		REPS ◯	REPS ◯	REPS ◯	REPS ◯	REPS ◯
BEST INCREASE ◀ WEIGHT ▶						
		REPS ◯	REPS ◯	REPS ◯	REPS ◯	REPS ◯
BEST INCREASE ◀ WEIGHT ▶						
		REPS ◯	REPS ◯	REPS ◯	REPS ◯	REPS ◯
BEST INCREASE ◀ WEIGHT ▶						
		REPS ◯	REPS ◯	REPS ◯	REPS ◯	REPS ◯
BEST INCREASE ◀ WEIGHT ▶						
		REPS ◯	REPS ◯	REPS ◯	REPS ◯	REPS ◯
BEST INCREASE ◀ WEIGHT ▶						

EXERCISE ——— SETS ——— REPS AND DONE! ———

	REPS ✓	REPS ✓	REPS ✓	REPS ✓	REPS ✓
BEST INCREASE — WEIGHT					
	REPS	REPS	REPS	REPS	REPS
BEST INCREASE — WEIGHT					
	REPS	REPS	REPS	REPS	REPS
BEST INCREASE — WEIGHT					
	REPS	REPS	REPS	REPS	REPS
BEST INCREASE — WEIGHT					
	REPS	REPS	REPS	REPS	REPS
BEST INCREASE — WEIGHT					
	REPS	REPS	REPS	REPS	REPS
BEST INCREASE — WEIGHT					
	REPS	REPS	REPS	REPS	REPS
BEST INCREASE — WEIGHT					
	REPS	REPS	REPS	REPS	REPS
BEST INCREASE — WEIGHT					
	REPS	REPS	REPS	REPS	REPS
BEST INCREASE — WEIGHT					
	REPS	REPS	REPS	REPS	REPS
BEST INCREASE — WEIGHT					
	REPS	REPS	REPS	REPS	REPS
BEST INCREASE — WEIGHT					
	REPS	REPS	REPS	REPS	REPS
BEST INCREASE — WEIGHT					

EXERCISE	SETS	REPS AND DONE!

		REPS ☐	REPS ☐	REPS ☐	REPS ☐	REPS ☐
BEST INCREASE WEIGHT						
		REPS ☐	REPS ☐	REPS ☐	REPS ☐	REPS ☐
BEST INCREASE WEIGHT						
		REPS ☐	REPS ☐	REPS ☐	REPS ☐	REPS ☐
BEST INCREASE WEIGHT						
		REPS ☐	REPS ☐	REPS ☐	REPS ☐	REPS ☐
BEST INCREASE WEIGHT						
		REPS ☐	REPS ☐	REPS ☐	REPS ☐	REPS ☐
BEST INCREASE WEIGHT						
		REPS ☐	REPS ☐	REPS ☐	REPS ☐	REPS ☐
BEST INCREASE WEIGHT						
		REPS ☐	REPS ☐	REPS ☐	REPS ☐	REPS ☐
BEST INCREASE WEIGHT						
		REPS ☐	REPS ☐	REPS ☐	REPS ☐	REPS ☐
BEST INCREASE WEIGHT						
		REPS ☐	REPS ☐	REPS ☐	REPS ☐	REPS ☐
BEST INCREASE WEIGHT						
		REPS ☐	REPS ☐	REPS ☐	REPS ☐	REPS ☐
BEST INCREASE WEIGHT						
		REPS ☐	REPS ☐	REPS ☐	REPS ☐	REPS ☐
BEST INCREASE WEIGHT						

EXERCISE ———— SETS ———— REPS AND DONE! ————

		REPS ✓	REPS ✓	REPS ✓	REPS ✓	REPS ✓
	BEST INCREASE → WEIGHT →					
		REPS	REPS	REPS	REPS	REPS
	BEST INCREASE → WEIGHT →					
		REPS	REPS	REPS	REPS	REPS
	BEST INCREASE → WEIGHT →					
		REPS	REPS	REPS	REPS	REPS
	BEST INCREASE → WEIGHT →					
		REPS	REPS	REPS	REPS	REPS
	BEST INCREASE → WEIGHT →					
		REPS	REPS	REPS	REPS	REPS
	BEST INCREASE → WEIGHT →					
		REPS	REPS	REPS	REPS	REPS
	BEST INCREASE → WEIGHT →					
		REPS	REPS	REPS	REPS	REPS
	BEST INCREASE → WEIGHT →					
		REPS	REPS	REPS	REPS	REPS
	BEST INCREASE → WEIGHT →					
		REPS	REPS	REPS	REPS	REPS
	BEST INCREASE → WEIGHT →					
		REPS	REPS	REPS	REPS	REPS
	BEST INCREASE → WEIGHT →					
		REPS	REPS	REPS	REPS	REPS
	BEST INCREASE → WEIGHT →					

		REPS ☐	REPS ☐	REPS ☐	REPS ☐	REPS ☐
BEST INCREASE ◄ WEIGHT ►						
		REPS ☐	REPS ☐	REPS ☐	REPS ☐	REPS ☐
BEST INCREASE ◄ WEIGHT ►						
		REPS ☐	REPS ☐	REPS ☐	REPS ☐	REPS ☐
BEST INCREASE ◄ WEIGHT ►						
		REPS ☐	REPS ☐	REPS ☐	REPS ☐	REPS ☐
BEST INCREASE ◄ WEIGHT ►						
		REPS ☐	REPS ☐	REPS ☐	REPS ☐	REPS ☐
BEST INCREASE ◄ WEIGHT ►						
		REPS ☐	REPS ☐	REPS ☐	REPS ☐	REPS ☐
BEST INCREASE ◄ WEIGHT ►						
		REPS ☐	REPS ☐	REPS ☐	REPS ☐	REPS ☐
BEST INCREASE ◄ WEIGHT ►						
		REPS ☐	REPS ☐	REPS ☐	REPS ☐	REPS ☐
BEST INCREASE ◄ WEIGHT ►						
		REPS ☐	REPS ☐	REPS ☐	REPS ☐	REPS ☐
BEST INCREASE ◄ WEIGHT ►						
		REPS ☐	REPS ☐	REPS ☐	REPS ☐	REPS ☐
BEST INCREASE ◄ WEIGHT ►						
		REPS ☐	REPS ☐	REPS ☐	REPS ☐	REPS ☐
BEST INCREASE ◄ WEIGHT ►						

EXERCISE — SETS — REPS AND DONE! —

		✔ REPS	✔ REPS	✔ REPS	✔ REPS	✔ REPS
BEST INCREASE — WEIGHT						
		REPS	REPS	REPS	REPS	REPS
BEST INCREASE — WEIGHT						
		REPS	REPS	REPS	REPS	REPS
BEST INCREASE — WEIGHT						
		REPS	REPS	REPS	REPS	REPS
BEST INCREASE — WEIGHT						
		REPS	REPS	REPS	REPS	REPS
BEST INCREASE — WEIGHT						
		REPS	REPS	REPS	REPS	REPS
BEST INCREASE — WEIGHT						
		REPS	REPS	REPS	REPS	REPS
BEST INCREASE — WEIGHT						
		REPS	REPS	REPS	REPS	REPS
BEST INCREASE — WEIGHT						
		REPS	REPS	REPS	REPS	REPS
BEST INCREASE — WEIGHT						
		REPS	REPS	REPS	REPS	REPS
BEST INCREASE — WEIGHT						
		REPS	REPS	REPS	REPS	REPS
BEST INCREASE — WEIGHT						
		REPS	REPS	REPS	REPS	REPS
BEST INCREASE — WEIGHT						

		REPS ☐	REPS ☐	REPS ☐	REPS ☐	REPS ☐
BEST INCREASE — WEIGHT						
		REPS ☐	REPS ☐	REPS ☐	REPS ☐	REPS ☐
BEST INCREASE — WEIGHT						
		REPS ☐	REPS ☐	REPS ☐	REPS ☐	REPS ☐
BEST INCREASE — WEIGHT						
		REPS ☐	REPS ☐	REPS ☐	REPS ☐	REPS ☐
BEST INCREASE — WEIGHT						
		REPS ☐	REPS ☐	REPS ☐	REPS ☐	REPS ☐
BEST INCREASE — WEIGHT						
		REPS ☐	REPS ☐	REPS ☐	REPS ☐	REPS ☐
BEST INCREASE — WEIGHT						
		REPS ☐	REPS ☐	REPS ☐	REPS ☐	REPS ☐
BEST INCREASE — WEIGHT						
		REPS ☐	REPS ☐	REPS ☐	REPS ☐	REPS ☐
BEST INCREASE — WEIGHT						
		REPS ☐	REPS ☐	REPS ☐	REPS ☐	REPS ☐
BEST INCREASE — WEIGHT						
		REPS ☐	REPS ☐	REPS ☐	REPS ☐	REPS ☐
BEST INCREASE — WEIGHT						

EXERCISE — SETS — REPS AND DONE! —

	REPS ✓	REPS ✓	REPS ✓	REPS ✓	REPS ✓
BEST INCREASE ◄ WEIGHT ►					
	REPS	REPS	REPS	REPS	REPS
BEST INCREASE ◄ WEIGHT ►					
	REPS	REPS	REPS	REPS	REPS
BEST INCREASE ◄ WEIGHT ►					
	REPS	REPS	REPS	REPS	REPS
BEST INCREASE ◄ WEIGHT ►					
	REPS	REPS	REPS	REPS	REPS
BEST INCREASE ◄ WEIGHT ►					
	REPS	REPS	REPS	REPS	REPS
BEST INCREASE ◄ WEIGHT ►					
	REPS	REPS	REPS	REPS	REPS
BEST INCREASE ◄ WEIGHT ►					
	REPS	REPS	REPS	REPS	REPS
BEST INCREASE ◄ WEIGHT ►					
	REPS	REPS	REPS	REPS	REPS
BEST INCREASE ◄ WEIGHT ►					
	REPS	REPS	REPS	REPS	REPS
BEST INCREASE ◄ WEIGHT ►					
	REPS	REPS	REPS	REPS	REPS
BEST INCREASE ◄ WEIGHT ►					

	REPS ☐	REPS ☐	REPS ☐	REPS ☐	REPS ☐
BEST INCREASE ◄ WEIGHT ►					
	REPS ☐	REPS ☐	REPS ☐	REPS ☐	REPS ☐
BEST INCREASE ◄ WEIGHT ►					
	REPS ☐	REPS ☐	REPS ☐	REPS ☐	REPS ☐
BEST INCREASE ◄ WEIGHT ►					
	REPS ☐	REPS ☐	REPS ☐	REPS ☐	REPS ☐
BEST INCREASE ◄ WEIGHT ►					
	REPS ☐	REPS ☐	REPS ☐	REPS ☐	REPS ☐
BEST INCREASE ◄ WEIGHT ►					
	REPS ☐	REPS ☐	REPS ☐	REPS ☐	REPS ☐
BEST INCREASE ◄ WEIGHT ►					
	REPS ☐	REPS ☐	REPS ☐	REPS ☐	REPS ☐
BEST INCREASE ◄ WEIGHT ►					
	REPS ☐	REPS ☐	REPS ☐	REPS ☐	REPS ☐
BEST INCREASE ◄ WEIGHT ►					
	REPS ☐	REPS ☐	REPS ☐	REPS ☐	REPS ☐
BEST INCREASE ◄ WEIGHT ►					
	REPS ☐	REPS ☐	REPS ☐	REPS ☐	REPS ☐
BEST INCREASE ◄ WEIGHT ►					

EXERCISE	SETS	REPS AND DONE!

		REPS ✓	REPS ✓	REPS ✓	REPS ✓	REPS ✓
BEST INCREASE → WEIGHT →						
		REPS	REPS	REPS	REPS	REPS
BEST INCREASE → WEIGHT →						
		REPS	REPS	REPS	REPS	REPS
BEST INCREASE → WEIGHT →						
		REPS	REPS	REPS	REPS	REPS
BEST INCREASE → WEIGHT →						
		REPS	REPS	REPS	REPS	REPS
BEST INCREASE → WEIGHT →						
		REPS	REPS	REPS	REPS	REPS
BEST INCREASE → WEIGHT →						
		REPS	REPS	REPS	REPS	REPS
BEST INCREASE → WEIGHT →						
		REPS	REPS	REPS	REPS	REPS
BEST INCREASE → WEIGHT →						
		REPS	REPS	REPS	REPS	REPS
BEST INCREASE → WEIGHT →						
		REPS	REPS	REPS	REPS	REPS
BEST INCREASE → WEIGHT →						
		REPS	REPS	REPS	REPS	REPS
BEST INCREASE → WEIGHT →						

EXERCISE ——— SETS ——— REPS AND DONE! ———

		REPS ☐	REPS ☐	REPS ☐	REPS ☐	REPS ☐
BEST INCREASE → WEIGHT →						
		REPS ☐	REPS ☐	REPS ☐	REPS ☐	REPS ☐
BEST INCREASE → WEIGHT →						
		REPS ☐	REPS ☐	REPS ☐	REPS ☐	REPS ☐
BEST INCREASE → WEIGHT →						
		REPS ☐	REPS ☐	REPS ☐	REPS ☐	REPS ☐
BEST INCREASE → WEIGHT →						
		REPS ☐	REPS ☐	REPS ☐	REPS ☐	REPS ☐
BEST INCREASE → WEIGHT →						
		REPS ☐	REPS ☐	REPS ☐	REPS ☐	REPS ☐
BEST INCREASE → WEIGHT →						
		REPS ☐	REPS ☐	REPS ☐	REPS ☐	REPS ☐
BEST INCREASE → WEIGHT →						
		REPS ☐	REPS ☐	REPS ☐	REPS ☐	REPS ☐
BEST INCREASE → WEIGHT →						
		REPS ☐	REPS ☐	REPS ☐	REPS ☐	REPS ☐
BEST INCREASE → WEIGHT →						
		REPS ☐	REPS ☐	REPS ☐	REPS ☐	REPS ☐
BEST INCREASE → WEIGHT →						

EXERCISE — SETS — REPS AND DONE!

	SETS	✓ REPS ☐	✓ REPS ☐	✓ REPS ☐	✓ REPS ☐	✓ REPS ☐
BEST INCREASE → WEIGHT						
		REPS ☐	REPS ☐	REPS ☐	REPS ☐	REPS ☐
BEST INCREASE → WEIGHT						
		REPS ☐	REPS ☐	REPS ☐	REPS ☐	REPS ☐
BEST INCREASE → WEIGHT						
		REPS ☐	REPS ☐	REPS ☐	REPS ☐	REPS ☐
BEST INCREASE → WEIGHT						
		REPS ☐	REPS ☐	REPS ☐	REPS ☐	REPS ☐
BEST INCREASE → WEIGHT						
		REPS ☐	REPS ☐	REPS ☐	REPS ☐	REPS ☐
BEST INCREASE → WEIGHT						
		REPS ☐	REPS ☐	REPS ☐	REPS ☐	REPS ☐
BEST INCREASE → WEIGHT						
		REPS ☐	REPS ☐	REPS ☐	REPS ☐	REPS ☐
BEST INCREASE → WEIGHT						
		REPS ☐	REPS ☐	REPS ☐	REPS ☐	REPS ☐
BEST INCREASE → WEIGHT						
		REPS ☐	REPS ☐	REPS ☐	REPS ☐	REPS ☐
BEST INCREASE → WEIGHT						
		REPS ☐	REPS ☐	REPS ☐	REPS ☐	REPS ☐
BEST INCREASE → WEIGHT						

EXERCISE ——— SETS ——— REPS AND DONE! ———

BEST INCREASE	WEIGHT	REPS ☐	REPS ☐	REPS ☐	REPS ☐	REPS ☐

BEST INCREASE	WEIGHT	REPS ☐	REPS ☐	REPS ☐	REPS ☐	REPS ☐

BEST INCREASE	WEIGHT	REPS ☐	REPS ☐	REPS ☐	REPS ☐	REPS ☐

BEST INCREASE	WEIGHT	REPS ☐	REPS ☐	REPS ☐	REPS ☐	REPS ☐

BEST INCREASE	WEIGHT	REPS ☐	REPS ☐	REPS ☐	REPS ☐	REPS ☐

BEST INCREASE	WEIGHT	REPS ☐	REPS ☐	REPS ☐	REPS ☐	REPS ☐

BEST INCREASE	WEIGHT	REPS ☐	REPS ☐	REPS ☐	REPS ☐	REPS ☐

BEST INCREASE	WEIGHT	REPS ☐	REPS ☐	REPS ☐	REPS ☐	REPS ☐

BEST INCREASE	WEIGHT	REPS ☐	REPS ☐	REPS ☐	REPS ☐	REPS ☐

BEST INCREASE	WEIGHT	REPS ☐	REPS ☐	REPS ☐	REPS ☐	REPS ☐

EXERCISE — SETS — REPS AND DONE!

	REPS ✓	REPS ✓	REPS ✓	REPS ✓	REPS ✓
BEST INCREASE — WEIGHT					
	REPS	REPS	REPS	REPS	REPS
BEST INCREASE — WEIGHT					
	REPS	REPS	REPS	REPS	REPS
BEST INCREASE — WEIGHT					
	REPS	REPS	REPS	REPS	REPS
BEST INCREASE — WEIGHT					
	REPS	REPS	REPS	REPS	REPS
BEST INCREASE — WEIGHT					
	REPS	REPS	REPS	REPS	REPS
BEST INCREASE — WEIGHT					
	REPS	REPS	REPS	REPS	REPS
BEST INCREASE — WEIGHT					
	REPS	REPS	REPS	REPS	REPS
BEST INCREASE — WEIGHT					
	REPS	REPS	REPS	REPS	REPS
BEST INCREASE — WEIGHT					
	REPS	REPS	REPS	REPS	REPS
BEST INCREASE — WEIGHT					
	REPS	REPS	REPS	REPS	REPS
BEST INCREASE — WEIGHT					
	REPS	REPS	REPS	REPS	REPS
BEST INCREASE — WEIGHT					

EXERCISE ———— SETS ———— REPS AND DONE! ————

EXERCISE	SETS	REPS ✓	REPS ✓	REPS ✓	REPS ✓	REPS ✓
BEST INCREASE — WEIGHT						
		REPS	REPS	REPS	REPS	REPS
BEST INCREASE — WEIGHT						
		REPS	REPS	REPS	REPS	REPS
BEST INCREASE — WEIGHT						
		REPS	REPS	REPS	REPS	REPS
BEST INCREASE — WEIGHT						
		REPS	REPS	REPS	REPS	REPS
BEST INCREASE — WEIGHT						
		REPS	REPS	REPS	REPS	REPS
BEST INCREASE — WEIGHT						
		REPS	REPS	REPS	REPS	REPS
BEST INCREASE — WEIGHT						
		REPS	REPS	REPS	REPS	REPS
BEST INCREASE — WEIGHT						
		REPS	REPS	REPS	REPS	REPS
BEST INCREASE — WEIGHT						
		REPS	REPS	REPS	REPS	REPS
BEST INCREASE — WEIGHT						

EXERCISE	SETS	REPS AND DONE!				
		REPS ☑	REPS ☑	REPS ☑	REPS ☑	REPS ☑
BEST INCREASE ◄ WEIGHT ►						
		REPS ☐	REPS ☐	REPS ☐	REPS ☐	REPS ☐
BEST INCREASE ◄ WEIGHT ►						
		REPS ☐	REPS ☐	REPS ☐	REPS ☐	REPS ☐
BEST INCREASE ◄ WEIGHT ►						
		REPS ☐	REPS ☐	REPS ☐	REPS ☐	REPS ☐
BEST INCREASE ◄ WEIGHT ►						
		REPS ☐	REPS ☐	REPS ☐	REPS ☐	REPS ☐
BEST INCREASE ◄ WEIGHT ►						
		REPS ☐	REPS ☐	REPS ☐	REPS ☐	REPS ☐
BEST INCREASE ◄ WEIGHT ►						
		REPS ☐	REPS ☐	REPS ☐	REPS ☐	REPS ☐
BEST INCREASE ◄ WEIGHT ►						
		REPS ☐	REPS ☐	REPS ☐	REPS ☐	REPS ☐
BEST INCREASE ◄ WEIGHT ►						
		REPS ☐	REPS ☐	REPS ☐	REPS ☐	REPS ☐
BEST INCREASE ◄ WEIGHT ►						
		REPS ☐	REPS ☐	REPS ☐	REPS ☐	REPS ☐
BEST INCREASE ◄ WEIGHT ►						
		REPS ☐	REPS ☐	REPS ☐	REPS ☐	REPS ☐
BEST INCREASE ◄ WEIGHT ►						

		✓	✓	✓	✓	✓
		REPS ⬭	REPS ⬭	REPS ⬭	REPS ⬭	REPS ⬭
	BEST INCREASE ◄ WEIGHT ►					
		REPS ⬭	REPS ⬭	REPS ⬭	REPS ⬭	REPS ⬭
	BEST INCREASE ◄ WEIGHT ►					
		REPS ⬭	REPS ⬭	REPS ⬭	REPS ⬭	REPS ⬭
	BEST INCREASE ◄ WEIGHT ►					
		REPS ⬭	REPS ⬭	REPS ⬭	REPS ⬭	REPS ⬭
	BEST INCREASE ◄ WEIGHT ►					
		REPS ⬭	REPS ⬭	REPS ⬭	REPS ⬭	REPS ⬭
	BEST INCREASE ◄ WEIGHT ►					
		REPS ⬭	REPS ⬭	REPS ⬭	REPS ⬭	REPS ⬭
	BEST INCREASE ◄ WEIGHT ►					
		REPS ⬭	REPS ⬭	REPS ⬭	REPS ⬭	REPS ⬭
	BEST INCREASE ◄ WEIGHT ►					
		REPS ⬭	REPS ⬭	REPS ⬭	REPS ⬭	REPS ⬭
	BEST INCREASE ◄ WEIGHT ►					
		REPS ⬭	REPS ⬭	REPS ⬭	REPS ⬭	REPS ⬭
	BEST INCREASE ◄ WEIGHT ►					
		REPS ⬭	REPS ⬭	REPS ⬭	REPS ⬭	REPS ⬭
	BEST INCREASE ◄ WEIGHT ►					
		REPS ⬭	REPS ⬭	REPS ⬭	REPS ⬭	REPS ⬭
	BEST INCREASE ◄ WEIGHT ►					

EXERCISE ——— • SETS • ——— REPS AND DONE! ———

		✓	✓	✓	✓	✓
		REPS ☐	REPS ☐	REPS ☐	REPS ☐	REPS ☐
BEST INCREASE ◄ WEIGHT ►						
		REPS ☐	REPS ☐	REPS ☐	REPS ☐	REPS ☐
BEST INCREASE ◄ WEIGHT ►						
		REPS ☐	REPS ☐	REPS ☐	REPS ☐	REPS ☐
BEST INCREASE ◄ WEIGHT ►						
		REPS ☐	REPS ☐	REPS ☐	REPS ☐	REPS ☐
BEST INCREASE ◄ WEIGHT ►						
		REPS ☐	REPS ☐	REPS ☐	REPS ☐	REPS ☐
BEST INCREASE ◄ WEIGHT ►						
		REPS ☐	REPS ☐	REPS ☐	REPS ☐	REPS ☐
BEST INCREASE ◄ WEIGHT ►						
		REPS ☐	REPS ☐	REPS ☐	REPS ☐	REPS ☐
BEST INCREASE ◄ WEIGHT ►						
		REPS ☐	REPS ☐	REPS ☐	REPS ☐	REPS ☐
BEST INCREASE ◄ WEIGHT ►						
		REPS ☐	REPS ☐	REPS ☐	REPS ☐	REPS ☐
BEST INCREASE ◄ WEIGHT ►						
		REPS ☐	REPS ☐	REPS ☐	REPS ☐	REPS ☐
BEST INCREASE ◄ WEIGHT ►						
		REPS ☐	REPS ☐	REPS ☐	REPS ☐	REPS ☐
BEST INCREASE ◄ WEIGHT ►						

EXERCISE ● SETS ●───── REPS AND DONE! ─────●

EXERCISE	SETS	REPS ✔	REPS ✔	REPS ✔	REPS ✔	REPS ✔
BEST INCREASE ◄ WEIGHT ►						
		REPS	REPS	REPS	REPS	REPS
BEST INCREASE ◄ WEIGHT ►						
		REPS	REPS	REPS	REPS	REPS
BEST INCREASE ◄ WEIGHT ►						
		REPS	REPS	REPS	REPS	REPS
BEST INCREASE ◄ WEIGHT ►						
		REPS	REPS	REPS	REPS	REPS
BEST INCREASE ◄ WEIGHT ►						
		REPS	REPS	REPS	REPS	REPS
BEST INCREASE ◄ WEIGHT ►						
		REPS	REPS	REPS	REPS	REPS
BEST INCREASE ◄ WEIGHT ►						
		REPS	REPS	REPS	REPS	REPS
BEST INCREASE ◄ WEIGHT ►						
		REPS	REPS	REPS	REPS	REPS
BEST INCREASE ◄ WEIGHT ►						
		REPS	REPS	REPS	REPS	REPS
BEST INCREASE ◄ WEIGHT ►						
		REPS	REPS	REPS	REPS	REPS
BEST INCREASE ◄ WEIGHT ►						

EXERCISE ———• SETS •——— REPS AND DONE! ———•

	✔ REPS	✔ REPS	✔ REPS	✔ REPS	✔ REPS
BEST INCREASE ← WEIGHT →					
	REPS	REPS	REPS	REPS	REPS
BEST INCREASE ← WEIGHT →					
	REPS	REPS	REPS	REPS	REPS
BEST INCREASE ← WEIGHT →					
	REPS	REPS	REPS	REPS	REPS
BEST INCREASE ← WEIGHT →					
	REPS	REPS	REPS	REPS	REPS
BEST INCREASE ← WEIGHT →					
	REPS	REPS	REPS	REPS	REPS
BEST INCREASE ← WEIGHT →					
	REPS	REPS	REPS	REPS	REPS
BEST INCREASE ← WEIGHT →					
	REPS	REPS	REPS	REPS	REPS
BEST INCREASE ← WEIGHT →					
	REPS	REPS	REPS	REPS	REPS
BEST INCREASE ← WEIGHT →					
	REPS	REPS	REPS	REPS	REPS
BEST INCREASE ← WEIGHT →					
	REPS	REPS	REPS	REPS	REPS
BEST INCREASE ← WEIGHT →					
	REPS	REPS	REPS	REPS	REPS
BEST INCREASE ← WEIGHT →					

EXERCISE ● SETS ● REPS AND DONE! ●

EXERCISE	SETS	REPS ☐	REPS ☐	REPS ☐	REPS ☐	REPS ☐
BEST INCREASE → WEIGHT →						
		REPS ☐	REPS ☐	REPS ☐	REPS ☐	REPS ☐
BEST INCREASE → WEIGHT →						
		REPS ☐	REPS ☐	REPS ☐	REPS ☐	REPS ☐
BEST INCREASE → WEIGHT →						
		REPS ☐	REPS ☐	REPS ☐	REPS ☐	REPS ☐
BEST INCREASE → WEIGHT →						
		REPS ☐	REPS ☐	REPS ☐	REPS ☐	REPS ☐
BEST INCREASE → WEIGHT →						
		REPS ☐	REPS ☐	REPS ☐	REPS ☐	REPS ☐
BEST INCREASE → WEIGHT →						
		REPS ☐	REPS ☐	REPS ☐	REPS ☐	REPS ☐
BEST INCREASE → WEIGHT →						
		REPS ☐	REPS ☐	REPS ☐	REPS ☐	REPS ☐
BEST INCREASE → WEIGHT →						
		REPS ☐	REPS ☐	REPS ☐	REPS ☐	REPS ☐
BEST INCREASE → WEIGHT →						
		REPS ☐	REPS ☐	REPS ☐	REPS ☐	REPS ☐
BEST INCREASE → WEIGHT →						
		REPS ☐	REPS ☐	REPS ☐	REPS ☐	REPS ☐
BEST INCREASE → WEIGHT →						

EXERCISE	SETS	REPS AND DONE!				
		REPS ✓	REPS ✓	REPS ✓	REPS ✓	REPS ✓
BEST INCREASE — WEIGHT —						
		REPS	REPS	REPS	REPS	REPS
BEST INCREASE — WEIGHT —						
		REPS	REPS	REPS	REPS	REPS
BEST INCREASE — WEIGHT —						
		REPS	REPS	REPS	REPS	REPS
BEST INCREASE — WEIGHT —						
		REPS	REPS	REPS	REPS	REPS
BEST INCREASE — WEIGHT —						
		REPS	REPS	REPS	REPS	REPS
BEST INCREASE — WEIGHT —						
		REPS	REPS	REPS	REPS	REPS
BEST INCREASE — WEIGHT —						
		REPS	REPS	REPS	REPS	REPS
BEST INCREASE — WEIGHT —						
		REPS	REPS	REPS	REPS	REPS
BEST INCREASE — WEIGHT —						
		REPS	REPS	REPS	REPS	REPS
BEST INCREASE — WEIGHT —						
		REPS	REPS	REPS	REPS	REPS
BEST INCREASE — WEIGHT —						
		REPS	REPS	REPS	REPS	REPS
BEST INCREASE — WEIGHT —						

EXERCISE — SETS — REPS AND DONE! —

		REPS ✓	REPS ✓	REPS ✓	REPS ✓	REPS ✓
BEST INCREASE → WEIGHT →						
		REPS	REPS	REPS	REPS	REPS
BEST INCREASE → WEIGHT →						
		REPS	REPS	REPS	REPS	REPS
BEST INCREASE → WEIGHT →						
		REPS	REPS	REPS	REPS	REPS
BEST INCREASE → WEIGHT →						
		REPS	REPS	REPS	REPS	REPS
BEST INCREASE → WEIGHT →						
		REPS	REPS	REPS	REPS	REPS
BEST INCREASE → WEIGHT →						
		REPS	REPS	REPS	REPS	REPS
BEST INCREASE → WEIGHT →						
		REPS	REPS	REPS	REPS	REPS
BEST INCREASE → WEIGHT →						
		REPS	REPS	REPS	REPS	REPS
BEST INCREASE → WEIGHT →						
		REPS	REPS	REPS	REPS	REPS
BEST INCREASE → WEIGHT →						
		REPS	REPS	REPS	REPS	REPS
BEST INCREASE → WEIGHT →						

EXERCISE ———• SETS •——— REPS AND DONE! ———•

		REPS ✔	REPS ✔	REPS ✔	REPS ✔	REPS ✔
BEST INCREASE WEIGHT						
		REPS	REPS	REPS	REPS	REPS
BEST INCREASE WEIGHT						
		REPS	REPS	REPS	REPS	REPS
BEST INCREASE WEIGHT						
		REPS	REPS	REPS	REPS	REPS
BEST INCREASE WEIGHT						
		REPS	REPS	REPS	REPS	REPS
BEST INCREASE WEIGHT						
		REPS	REPS	REPS	REPS	REPS
BEST INCREASE WEIGHT						
		REPS	REPS	REPS	REPS	REPS
BEST INCREASE WEIGHT						
		REPS	REPS	REPS	REPS	REPS
BEST INCREASE WEIGHT						
		REPS	REPS	REPS	REPS	REPS
BEST INCREASE WEIGHT						
		REPS	REPS	REPS	REPS	REPS
BEST INCREASE WEIGHT						
		REPS	REPS	REPS	REPS	REPS
BEST INCREASE WEIGHT						

EXERCISE	SETS	REPS AND DONE!				
		REPS ☐	REPS ☐	REPS ☐	REPS ☐	REPS ☐
BEST INCREASE — WEIGHT						
		REPS ☐	REPS ☐	REPS ☐	REPS ☐	REPS ☐
BEST INCREASE — WEIGHT						
		REPS ☐	REPS ☐	REPS ☐	REPS ☐	REPS ☐
BEST INCREASE — WEIGHT						
		REPS ☐	REPS ☐	REPS ☐	REPS ☐	REPS ☐
BEST INCREASE — WEIGHT						
		REPS ☐	REPS ☐	REPS ☐	REPS ☐	REPS ☐
BEST INCREASE — WEIGHT						
		REPS ☐	REPS ☐	REPS ☐	REPS ☐	REPS ☐
BEST INCREASE — WEIGHT						
		REPS ☐	REPS ☐	REPS ☐	REPS ☐	REPS ☐
BEST INCREASE — WEIGHT						
		REPS ☐	REPS ☐	REPS ☐	REPS ☐	REPS ☐
BEST INCREASE — WEIGHT						
		REPS ☐	REPS ☐	REPS ☐	REPS ☐	REPS ☐
BEST INCREASE — WEIGHT						
		REPS ☐	REPS ☐	REPS ☐	REPS ☐	REPS ☐
BEST INCREASE — WEIGHT						
		REPS ☐	REPS ☐	REPS ☐	REPS ☐	REPS ☐
BEST INCREASE — WEIGHT						

EXERCISE ———• SETS •——— REPS AND DONE! ———•

		✓	✓	✓	✓	✓
		REPS	REPS	REPS	REPS	REPS
BEST INCREASE — WEIGHT						
		REPS	REPS	REPS	REPS	REPS
BEST INCREASE — WEIGHT						
		REPS	REPS	REPS	REPS	REPS
BEST INCREASE — WEIGHT						
		REPS	REPS	REPS	REPS	REPS
BEST INCREASE — WEIGHT						
		REPS	REPS	REPS	REPS	REPS
BEST INCREASE — WEIGHT						
		REPS	REPS	REPS	REPS	REPS
BEST INCREASE — WEIGHT						
		REPS	REPS	REPS	REPS	REPS
BEST INCREASE — WEIGHT						
		REPS	REPS	REPS	REPS	REPS
BEST INCREASE — WEIGHT						
		REPS	REPS	REPS	REPS	REPS
BEST INCREASE — WEIGHT						
		REPS	REPS	REPS	REPS	REPS
BEST INCREASE — WEIGHT						
		REPS	REPS	REPS	REPS	REPS
BEST INCREASE — WEIGHT						
		REPS	REPS	REPS	REPS	REPS
BEST INCREASE — WEIGHT						

			REPS ✓	REPS ✓	REPS ✓	REPS ✓	REPS ✓
	BEST INCREASE ◄ WEIGHT ►						
			REPS	REPS	REPS	REPS	REPS
	BEST INCREASE ◄ WEIGHT ►						
			REPS	REPS	REPS	REPS	REPS
	BEST INCREASE ◄ WEIGHT ►						
			REPS	REPS	REPS	REPS	REPS
	BEST INCREASE ◄ WEIGHT ►						
			REPS	REPS	REPS	REPS	REPS
	BEST INCREASE ◄ WEIGHT ►						
			REPS	REPS	REPS	REPS	REPS
	BEST INCREASE ◄ WEIGHT ►						
			REPS	REPS	REPS	REPS	REPS
	BEST INCREASE ◄ WEIGHT ►						
			REPS	REPS	REPS	REPS	REPS
	BEST INCREASE ◄ WEIGHT ►						
			REPS	REPS	REPS	REPS	REPS
	BEST INCREASE ◄ WEIGHT ►						
			REPS	REPS	REPS	REPS	REPS
	BEST INCREASE ◄ WEIGHT ►						
			REPS	REPS	REPS	REPS	REPS
	BEST INCREASE ◄ WEIGHT ►						

	REPS ✓	REPS ✓	REPS ✓	REPS ✓	REPS ✓
BEST INCREASE ← WEIGHT					
	REPS	REPS	REPS	REPS	REPS
BEST INCREASE ← WEIGHT					
	REPS	REPS	REPS	REPS	REPS
BEST INCREASE ← WEIGHT					
	REPS	REPS	REPS	REPS	REPS
BEST INCREASE ← WEIGHT					
	REPS	REPS	REPS	REPS	REPS
BEST INCREASE ← WEIGHT					
	REPS	REPS	REPS	REPS	REPS
BEST INCREASE ← WEIGHT					
	REPS	REPS	REPS	REPS	REPS
BEST INCREASE ← WEIGHT					
	REPS	REPS	REPS	REPS	REPS
BEST INCREASE ← WEIGHT					
	REPS	REPS	REPS	REPS	REPS
BEST INCREASE ← WEIGHT					
	REPS	REPS	REPS	REPS	REPS
BEST INCREASE ← WEIGHT					
	REPS	REPS	REPS	REPS	REPS
BEST INCREASE ← WEIGHT					
	REPS	REPS	REPS	REPS	REPS
BEST INCREASE ← WEIGHT					

EXERCISE — SETS — REPS AND DONE! —

	REPS ☑	REPS ☑	REPS ☑	REPS ☑	REPS ☑
BEST INCREASE — WEIGHT					
	REPS ☐	REPS ☐	REPS ☐	REPS ☐	REPS ☐
BEST INCREASE — WEIGHT					
	REPS ☐	REPS ☐	REPS ☐	REPS ☐	REPS ☐
BEST INCREASE — WEIGHT					
	REPS ☐	REPS ☐	REPS ☐	REPS ☐	REPS ☐
BEST INCREASE — WEIGHT					
	REPS ☐	REPS ☐	REPS ☐	REPS ☐	REPS ☐
BEST INCREASE — WEIGHT					
	REPS ☐	REPS ☐	REPS ☐	REPS ☐	REPS ☐
BEST INCREASE — WEIGHT					
	REPS ☐	REPS ☐	REPS ☐	REPS ☐	REPS ☐
BEST INCREASE — WEIGHT					
	REPS ☐	REPS ☐	REPS ☐	REPS ☐	REPS ☐
BEST INCREASE — WEIGHT					
	REPS ☐	REPS ☐	REPS ☐	REPS ☐	REPS ☐
BEST INCREASE — WEIGHT					
	REPS ☐	REPS ☐	REPS ☐	REPS ☐	REPS ☐
BEST INCREASE — WEIGHT					
	REPS ☐	REPS ☐	REPS ☐	REPS ☐	REPS ☐
BEST INCREASE — WEIGHT					

	REPS ✔	REPS ✔	REPS ✔	REPS ✔	REPS ✔
BEST INCREASE ◄ WEIGHT ►					
	REPS	REPS	REPS	REPS	REPS
BEST INCREASE ◄ WEIGHT ►					
	REPS	REPS	REPS	REPS	REPS
BEST INCREASE ◄ WEIGHT ►					
	REPS	REPS	REPS	REPS	REPS
BEST INCREASE ◄ WEIGHT ►					
	REPS	REPS	REPS	REPS	REPS
BEST INCREASE ◄ WEIGHT ►					
	REPS	REPS	REPS	REPS	REPS
BEST INCREASE ◄ WEIGHT ►					
	REPS	REPS	REPS	REPS	REPS
BEST INCREASE ◄ WEIGHT ►					
	REPS	REPS	REPS	REPS	REPS
BEST INCREASE ◄ WEIGHT ►					
	REPS	REPS	REPS	REPS	REPS
BEST INCREASE ◄ WEIGHT ►					
	REPS	REPS	REPS	REPS	REPS
BEST INCREASE ◄ WEIGHT ►					
	REPS	REPS	REPS	REPS	REPS
BEST INCREASE ◄ WEIGHT ►					

EXERCISE ———— • SETS • ———— REPS AND DONE! ————•

EXERCISE	SETS	REPS	REPS	REPS	REPS	REPS
		REPS ⬜	REPS ⬜	REPS ⬜	REPS ⬜	REPS ⬜
BEST INCREASE ◄ WEIGHT ►						
		REPS ⬜	REPS ⬜	REPS ⬜	REPS ⬜	REPS ⬜
BEST INCREASE ◄ WEIGHT ►						
		REPS ⬜	REPS ⬜	REPS ⬜	REPS ⬜	REPS ⬜
BEST INCREASE ◄ WEIGHT ►						
		REPS ⬜	REPS ⬜	REPS ⬜	REPS ⬜	REPS ⬜
BEST INCREASE ◄ WEIGHT ►						
		REPS ⬜	REPS ⬜	REPS ⬜	REPS ⬜	REPS ⬜
BEST INCREASE ◄ WEIGHT ►						
		REPS ⬜	REPS ⬜	REPS ⬜	REPS ⬜	REPS ⬜
BEST INCREASE ◄ WEIGHT ►						
		REPS ⬜	REPS ⬜	REPS ⬜	REPS ⬜	REPS ⬜
BEST INCREASE ◄ WEIGHT ►						
		REPS ⬜	REPS ⬜	REPS ⬜	REPS ⬜	REPS ⬜
BEST INCREASE ◄ WEIGHT ►						
		REPS ⬜	REPS ⬜	REPS ⬜	REPS ⬜	REPS ⬜
BEST INCREASE ◄ WEIGHT ►						
		REPS ⬜	REPS ⬜	REPS ⬜	REPS ⬜	REPS ⬜
BEST INCREASE ◄ WEIGHT ►						
		REPS ⬜	REPS ⬜	REPS ⬜	REPS ⬜	REPS ⬜
BEST INCREASE ◄ WEIGHT ►						

EXERCISE	SETS	REPS AND DONE!
		REPS ✓ REPS ✓ REPS ✓ REPS ✓ REPS ✓
BEST INCREASE → WEIGHT →		
		REPS ☐ REPS ☐ REPS ☐ REPS ☐ REPS ☐
BEST INCREASE → WEIGHT →		
		REPS ☐ REPS ☐ REPS ☐ REPS ☐ REPS ☐
BEST INCREASE → WEIGHT →		
		REPS ☐ REPS ☐ REPS ☐ REPS ☐ REPS ☐
BEST INCREASE → WEIGHT →		
		REPS ☐ REPS ☐ REPS ☐ REPS ☐ REPS ☐
BEST INCREASE → WEIGHT →		
		REPS ☐ REPS ☐ REPS ☐ REPS ☐ REPS ☐
BEST INCREASE → WEIGHT →		
		REPS ☐ REPS ☐ REPS ☐ REPS ☐ REPS ☐
BEST INCREASE → WEIGHT →		
		REPS ☐ REPS ☐ REPS ☐ REPS ☐ REPS ☐
BEST INCREASE → WEIGHT →		
		REPS ☐ REPS ☐ REPS ☐ REPS ☐ REPS ☐
BEST INCREASE → WEIGHT →		
		REPS ☐ REPS ☐ REPS ☐ REPS ☐ REPS ☐
BEST INCREASE → WEIGHT →		
		REPS ☐ REPS ☐ REPS ☐ REPS ☐ REPS ☐
BEST INCREASE → WEIGHT →		
		REPS ☐ REPS ☐ REPS ☐ REPS ☐ REPS ☐
BEST INCREASE → WEIGHT →		

EXERCISE ——— SETS ——— REPS AND DONE! ———

		REPS ☐	REPS ☐	REPS ☐	REPS ☐	REPS ☐
BEST INCREASE ← WEIGHT →						
		REPS ☐	REPS ☐	REPS ☐	REPS ☐	REPS ☐
BEST INCREASE ← WEIGHT →						
		REPS ☐	REPS ☐	REPS ☐	REPS ☐	REPS ☐
BEST INCREASE ← WEIGHT →						
		REPS ☐	REPS ☐	REPS ☐	REPS ☐	REPS ☐
BEST INCREASE ← WEIGHT →						
		REPS ☐	REPS ☐	REPS ☐	REPS ☐	REPS ☐
BEST INCREASE ← WEIGHT →						
		REPS ☐	REPS ☐	REPS ☐	REPS ☐	REPS ☐
BEST INCREASE ← WEIGHT →						
		REPS ☐	REPS ☐	REPS ☐	REPS ☐	REPS ☐
BEST INCREASE ← WEIGHT →						
		REPS ☐	REPS ☐	REPS ☐	REPS ☐	REPS ☐
BEST INCREASE ← WEIGHT →						
		REPS ☐	REPS ☐	REPS ☐	REPS ☐	REPS ☐
BEST INCREASE ← WEIGHT →						
		REPS ☐	REPS ☐	REPS ☐	REPS ☐	REPS ☐
BEST INCREASE ← WEIGHT →						
		REPS ☐	REPS ☐	REPS ☐	REPS ☐	REPS ☐
BEST INCREASE ← WEIGHT →						

EXERCISE ———— SETS ———— REPS AND DONE! ————

		REPS ✓	REPS ✓	REPS ✓	REPS ✓	REPS ✓
BEST INCREASE → WEIGHT						
		REPS	REPS	REPS	REPS	REPS
BEST INCREASE → WEIGHT						
		REPS	REPS	REPS	REPS	REPS
BEST INCREASE → WEIGHT						
		REPS	REPS	REPS	REPS	REPS
BEST INCREASE → WEIGHT						
		REPS	REPS	REPS	REPS	REPS
BEST INCREASE → WEIGHT						
		REPS	REPS	REPS	REPS	REPS
BEST INCREASE → WEIGHT						
		REPS	REPS	REPS	REPS	REPS
BEST INCREASE → WEIGHT						
		REPS	REPS	REPS	REPS	REPS
BEST INCREASE → WEIGHT						
		REPS	REPS	REPS	REPS	REPS
BEST INCREASE → WEIGHT						
		REPS	REPS	REPS	REPS	REPS
BEST INCREASE → WEIGHT						
		REPS	REPS	REPS	REPS	REPS
BEST INCREASE → WEIGHT						

www.ingramcontent.com/pod-product-compliance
Lightning Source LLC
Chambersburg PA
CBHW070212290526
45789CB00002B/972